WORKOUT FOR SENIORS OVER 60
3 BOOKS IN 1

150 Illustrated Exercises To Improve Strength, Balance And Flexibility. Boost Your Confidence, Improve Your Quality Of Life and Regains A Renewed Youthfulness

DANIEL LINCOLN

IMPORTANT, READ CAREFULLY

DISCLAIMER: THIS BOOK DOES NOT PROVIDE MEDICAL ADVICE

This book contains information for general guidance only, including, but not limited to, written content, images, photos, and other items. Nothing in this book is meant to be a replacement for qualified medical guidance, diagnosis, or treatment. Never dismiss expert medical advice or put off getting it because of something you have read on this book; instead, always seek it out right away if you have any questions about a medical condition or treatment from your doctor or another trained healthcare practitioner. The execution of the exercises in this book is not the author's responsibility. The reader is alone in charge of their actions.

"To everyone who never gives up…"

Introduction

As we age, our strength, balance, and flexibility decline. Because of this, many older people embrace an unhealthy life. However, this inactivity merely accelerates physical aging and reduces flexibility. Why not try a workout, a diverse exercise created to improve the physical abilities required for daily activities to stay active and independent?

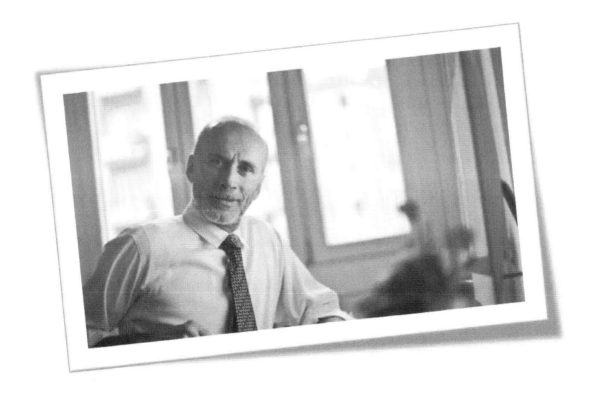

What is aging?

Aging is defined as "the decrease in an organism's functions with time, which results in a transformation of the body's organs." Functional training makes it feasible to remain active well into old age. Seniors can develop the muscles necessary for flexibility in daily activities by performing resistance exercises. Each person has a different path toward old age. However, they agree that keeping or re-discovering old abilities is important. Functional training, which consists of resistance exercises to overcome physical inactivity, is one method for doing this. Seniors who exercise find it simpler to go about their everyday lives, maintain a healthy weight, support emotional well-being, build immune systems, improve memory, and lessen stress. Workout is seen as a component of healthy aging.

What does workout mean?

Workout is a type of exercise that helps older persons become fitter and energized by having them perform exercises that simulate daily tasks.

Age makes it harder and harder to carry out various regular chores. The causes are osteoarthritis, muscular degeneration, and the pain it causes.

For instance, carrying groceries from the car to the house and then putting them away in the cabinets takes some arm strength and a minimum of body balance and shoulder flexibility. The goal of workouts for older persons is to improve balance, body strength, endurance, and joint flexibility. A combination of all these physical skills is needed for the majority of daily tasks. Older individuals must exercise all of their arm muscles to increase their ability to move objects and raise them to different heights. Additionally, they require the power to lift something and the dexterity to maneuver about without falling. In this case, performing a simple house workout or exercise will help improve seniors' flexibility in their aging process.

6 Mistakes To Avoid For Safety During Exercise

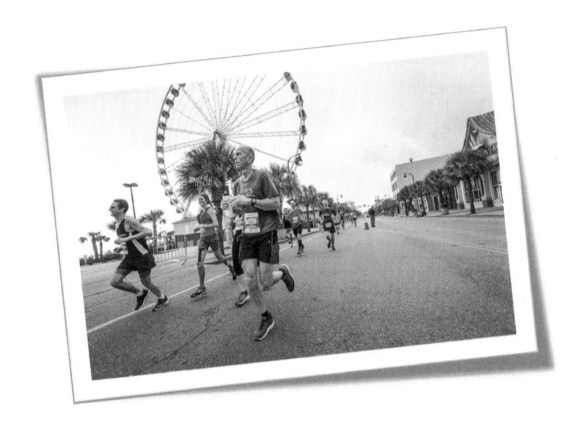

Starting an exercise routine is one of the top activities you can do to improve your health. You'll have more energy, be better able to engage in daily activities, and lower your risk of contracting chronic illnesses like diabetes and heart disease.

The two most important steps are knowing what you want to accomplish and creating a plan to get there. While any exercise is preferable to none, ensuring your workout is beneficial is crucial. After all, improper form during training may prevent you from gaining the advantages of movement or may increase your risk of injury.

Here are seven typical fitness mistakes people make and how to avoid them:

1.Excessive exercise It's usual for new exercisers to overdo it right away in today's "all or nothing" society.

Even people who last exercised in years trying to run a half-marathon without training. Try to push through it, and you'll pay for it later with an injury or the incapacity to engage in activities you'd like to.

What to do: Pay attention to your body's signals and allow it to relax and heal.

2.Using incorrect syntax.

Use perfect form when exercising, whether running, lifting weights, or doing a yoga routine, to obtain the desired results and reduce your chance of injury.

What to do: Schedule a few sessions with a personal trainer or make sure you're carrying out the exercises correctly.

3.Avoid warming up or cooling down.

In particular, if you're taking part in high-intensity activities, warming up before exercise helps your body prepare for physical activity and helps prevent injuries, missing heartbeats, and early weariness. The process of cooling down speeds up recovery and reduces muscular discomfort.

What to do: Before a workout, concentrate on dynamic warm-ups that involve movement, such as brisk walking, arm circles, marching in place, or jumping jacks. Any easy exercise that makes you sweat and warms your muscles is beneficial. Just concentrate on the body parts and muscles needed for your exercise. Static stretches that you hold for at least 30 seconds are good cool-down exercises.

4.Continually do the same exercise.

Not mixing up your activities can eventually result in fatigue or damage. However, any action is preferable to none.

Good for you if you enjoy jogging; you're active. But it makes sense to occasionally deviate from your regular schedule if your objective is to increase your general fitness.

How to ensure you're fit enough to do the things you want to do later in life: include various exercise types. This entails engaging in aerobic exercise, strengthening your muscles through weight training, and maintaining the flexibility of your muscles and joints with stretching and flexibility exercises.

5.Forgoing weightlifting.

Strength exercise is essential for maintaining muscle tone and developing powerful muscles. Weightlifting and resistance training develop strong connective tissues while enhancing strength and elasticity (ligaments and tendons). Strength training will help you accomplish daily activities from a biomechanical standpoint. Plus, strength training speeds up your metabolism, making it a great strategy to lose extra body fat.

What to do: Lifting weights is optional for resistance training. Strong muscles can be developed through yoga, swimming, and body weight exercises like lunges, push-ups, and workouts with resistance bands.

6.Ignoring the need for rest and recovery.

You need to obtain enough sleep for a workout to be lastingly effective. Your requirement for recovery will increase as your workout intensity increases.

What to do: Take a step back if you feel like you're doing too much too soon. It's acceptable to move slowly and take your time. After a workout, replacing lost calories and fluids is also critical. After working out, think about eating and drinking a liter of water.

7 Myths Of Physical Exercise

In light of the most recent research findings, we can debunk misconceptions about aging and exercise and alter our perspective on it. Let's examine seven aging and physical exercise myths in more detail:

1.Weakness, frailty, and dependence are inevitable side effects of aging.

The steady loss of muscle mass and strength that occurs with aging can be slowed or prevented by engaging in regular physical activity, especially after age 60.

In addition, most healthy elderly persons can continue to be independent in their everyday activities despite these changes and live without weakness.

2.Those that are older should minimize their physical activity:

This myth is still prevalent in some societies and among some older individuals (and younger people). Numerous studies have demonstrated that specific forms of exercise can help with most health issues. Remembering exercise is crucial for preventing several ailments is also vital.

3.Never again will I be as agile as I once was.

Truth: As you get older, your body changes. Your metabolism, muscle mass, hormones, and bone density could all vary. However, your power and performance level may definitely fall as you age. But you can still enjoy the health advantages and sense of success that come with working out. It's recommended to start slowly and adjust your exercises to your age-appropriate lifestyle goals. Remember that sitting down a lot is more detrimental than beneficial.

4.The chance of falling rises during exercise.

The truth is that regular exercise can help grow muscle, increase strength and endurance, and stop the loss of bone mass. Your balance will consequently get better, lowering your danger of falling. Exercises that improve balance should be a part of every senior's exercise program.

5.I am too old

There is no such thing as getting too old to exercise. It is always possible to start exercising and enhancing your general well-being. Compared to younger people, those who start being active later in life benefit more physically and mentally. It's recommended to begin with gentle and simple exercises and build up if you haven't tried exercising before or if it has been a while since you last did.

6.I shouldn't work out because I have arthritis and joint pain.

You should always exercise even if you have a chronic disease like arthritis. Quite often, the opposite is true. The effects or risk factors of diabetes, heart disease, and even cancer can be reduced by exercise.

7.Exercise can no longer improve my health because it is too late.

One of the most typical myths is this one. As long as possible, exercise can benefit both the body and the mind, stop the onset or aggravation of chronic illnesses, and improve overall health. According to studies, even those who are 90 years old and reside in nursing homes might gain advantages from regular exercise to increase their muscle power. Older individuals can also benefit from taking daily, easy walks or cycling.

Everyone should exercise. However, before starting any exercise, speak with your doctor or the rest of your healthcare team. They'll recommend a respectable personal trainer, or they might provide you with the appropriate workouts.

The Science Behind The Physical Workout

Recent studies have also demonstrated pretty convincingly the benefits of exercise, which include some very important benefits like lowering the risk of developing dementia.

Here are some reasons why science suggests we should continue working out, even if we don't necessarily enjoy it.

1.   This is significant because inflammation may be the root cause of various illnesses and mental disorders. C-reactive protein (CRP) and interleukin-6 (IL-6) are two inflammatory indicators that exercise is known to lower and are associated with various disorders. "The interesting thing about exercise is that it affects many organs and systems. Exercise's anti-inflammatory properties are probably one of the mechanisms underlying its protective effects against disorders, including cardiovascular disease, diabetes, some malignancies, and neurological diseases. As exercise is connected to changes in the secretion of stress hormones like epinephrine (also known as adrenaline) and norepinephrine, a new study demonstrates that a 20-minute moderate workout has detectable impacts on the immune system. Since hormone levels essentially return to baseline after you exercise, a rare workout won't replace it; you need to work out frequently. You want to harness the influence that accrues over time by getting active at least a couple of times per week.

1.   Reduces the risk of experiencing a heart attack and a stroke:

Even while inflammation plays a role in several cardiovascular effects of exercise, they merit their own category. Exercise is one of the healthiest things we can do for our hearts, which benefits blood pressure and cholesterol markers as well as the physical makeup of the heart and blood vessel function. While some studies claim that 30 minutes a day is sufficient to maintain heart health, others argue that more exercise is necessary to have a significant impact.

2.   Reduced chance of dementia

This could be the best argument in favor of exercising. Exercisers have been proven to have a considerably lower risk of dementia, including Alzheimer's disease. In contrast to non-exercisers, brain volume can increase over time for persons who start exercising somewhat late in life, as can test results for memory (their brains shrunk over time, which is a normal part of aging). Being physically active as we age can help with cognitive function and lower the risk of developing diseases like dementia and Alzheimer's. Exercise has a favorable impact on the hippocampus by increasing synaptic plasticity and the strength of nerve impulses in the brain.

Simple Workout Equipment For Seniors

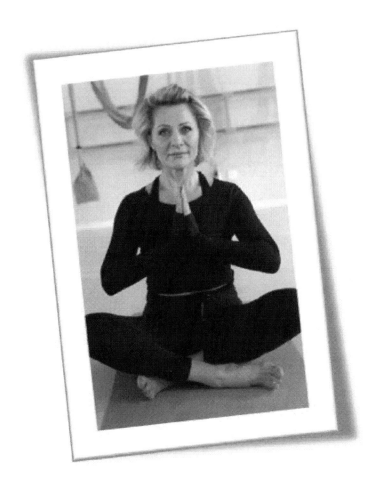

Selecting exercise equipment that is effective, entertaining, and safe for elders might be challenging. Various excellent options for seniors-friendly exercise equipment will help you burn calories, increase your heart rate, gain flexibility, and enhance your physical stamina! Here are some excellent examples of seniors workout equipment:

1. Stability Ball:

Core stability is essential for posture, balance, and standing. Seniors benefit greatly from simply sitting on a stability ball to strengthen their core muscles. With the ball, you can perform a variety of additional workouts, including stretches, to increase flexibility. The stability ball has various benefits for improving seniors' overall physical health.

2. Yoga mat

The ability to practice various low-impact movements on their feet, knees or while lying on the ground makes a yoga mat an excellent fitness gear for seniors. Pilates and yoga stretching routines frequently involve the usage of yoga mats. These are excellent seniors exercise options since they help seniors strengthen their core and improve their balance, making them safer when exercising and performing daily tasks.

3. Wrist Weights

Wrist weights can be used by seniors who want to increase their difficulty level while walking, running, using an elliptical machine, etc. If they choose, they can hold the weights in their hands instead of having them attached to their wrists.

These weights are relatively light—between one and three pounds—so they provide just the right amount of weight to make things more complicated without exerting too much pressure on their wrists.

4. Elliptical

Seniors who can stand for extended periods can burn some calories, enhance balance, and increase endurance by using an elliptical machine. The elliptical is a cross between walking and cross-country skiing but without the added impact. The arm levers that are incorporated provide seniors with a safety feature to grip onto and an additional muscular workout. Increased heart rate and more muscle growth are both possible with adjustable resistance. It's a fantastic machine all around for seniors.

5. Sitting Stepper

The mobility of your feet and legs can be improved by using a portable device known as a sitting stepper. The activity decreases serious vein thrombosis risk, which improves blood circulation, lessens stiffness, and is performed on a stationary machine.

Cautions For Individuals With Special Case

While regular exercise is beneficial for everyone, certain persons might need to take additional safety measures. Find the best workout program for you by asking your doctor for assistance if you have specific health issues. While exercising, if you experience any of the following, carefully slow down before stopping:

- **Dizzy or faint**
- **Nauseated**
- **Chest discomfort or stiffness**
- **Struggling to breathe**
- **Muscle control loss**

Arthritis: Running, jogging, jumping rope, or any exercise involving simultaneously lifting both feet off the ground, such as high-impact aerobics, should be avoided if you have arthritis that affects your joints.

Hot yoga is a popular new kind of exercise, sometimes referred to as Bikram yoga. Before beginning this style of yoga, those with arthritis should see their doctor.

People with arthritis may want to avoid hot yoga because heat can induce edema.

Osteoporosis: Jumping, running, or jogging can cause fractures in already-weakened bones. Always try to avoid abrupt, quick movements. Pick workouts that need to be controlled, slow movement. However, if you are normally strong and active with osteoporosis, you can perform slightly more impactful activity than someone who is fragile.

Diabetes:·

- Check your blood sugar levels before working out. Have a carbohydrate snack if the readings are under 100 mg/dl to avoid hypoglycemia. Start your activity only when the levels fall below 250 mg/dl if they are above that level.
- Always travel with someone who can assist you if your blood sugar levels fall. If a companion is not accessible, you should wear an identification that states that you have diabetes so that onlookers can assist you in the event of any unforeseen circumstances.

- ·Carry quick-acting carbohydrates in case you experience hypoglycemia, such as glucose pills.
- ·Exercise should be avoided if you have an infection since it may raise your blood sugar levels.

7 Benefits Of Workout For Seniors

1.   Increase in muscle mass.

Like younger people, exercise helps older people build strength and muscle mass. Stronger and bigger muscles better absorb a major fall's impact.

A senior with powerful arms can catch themselves and avoid having their head touch the ground. Strong muscles also safeguard bones and joints, lowering the possibility of suffering a significant injury in the event of a fall.

2.   It Improves mental capacity.

Regular exercisers typically have improved cognitive abilities. Specific neurotransmitters that support brain health, even under stress, are produced when you exercise. Regular exercise can improve cognitive function, making it easier for people to handle challenging circumstances and even prevent falls by keeping them away from potentially hazardous situations.

3.   Improve the quality of your sleep.

Regular workout among elders is associated with improved sleep and deeper slumber, which is important for seniors with unpredictable sleep patterns.

Exercise makes the body aware of the time of day and aids in maintaining a healthy circadian rhythm in seniors citizens. Problems with the circadian clock can cause irritability and lingering mental fog. Exercise outside and sunbathing are two benefits for seniors who need an excuse to be outside during the day.

4.   Enhanced reflexes

Because of their strong responses, younger people avoid falling more often than older people, whose reflexes decrease with age. Exercise can significantly increase reaction time by fostering speedier performance and muscle strength. People can avoid falling if they have rapid reflexes that enable them to grip something solid or lean against a wall immediately.

5.   Having healthy bones and preventing osteoporosis

Bones can become stronger through weight-bearing and resistance exercises.

The periosteum, or the outer layer of bone tissue, is gently pulled during contraction by the ligaments that join the muscles to the bones, increasing the density of the bone. Denser bones are less prone to fracture even after a fall.

6.   Effective coordination

Coordination is something that many people take for granted, just like balance. A person with good coordination may be able to roll after falling rather than crashing. An older person with good balance can fall and miss banging their head on a neighboring table corner. Coordination frequently happens unconsciously and automatically. Instead, it is the outcome of coordination training through consistent exercise.

7.   It decreased the chance of falling.

Overall, exercise's many physical advantages lead to a lower chance of falling. Regular workout benefits a person's overall health, but it's important also to consider how much less likely they are to fall and how likely they are to get hurt if they do.

The effects of injuries can be quite detrimental to elders' health, but the best way to avoid falls is for seniors to practice balance-related exercises on a daily basis. Additional health benefits and an overall improvement in quality of life will result from these workouts.

In this book, we will discuss three exercise phases for seniors to encourage good health, sickness-free, and long life span.

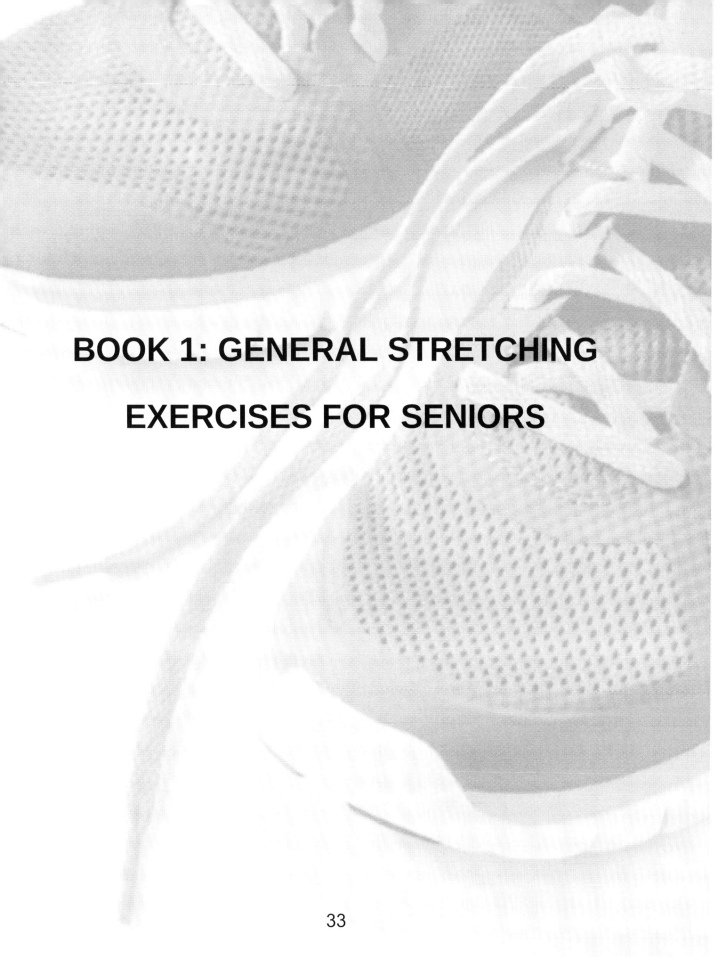

BOOK 1: GENERAL STRETCHING EXERCISES FOR SENIORS

Stretching has several advantages. They mainly help with pre- and post-exercise recuperation (post-stretching) and mobility, which is crucial for performance and ensures the preservation of health. After-activity regeneration techniques aim to ease muscle tension.

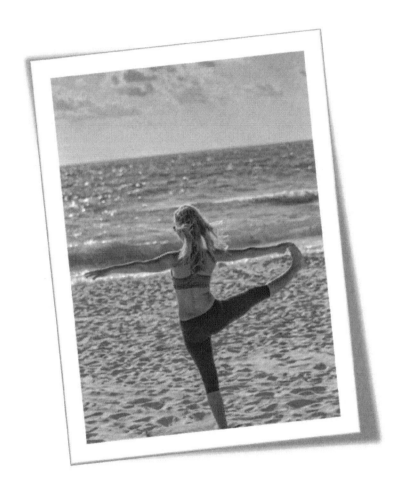

Even though stretching is largely static, it helps with mental healing. The purpose of stretching is to increase flexibility, range of motion, body balance, and recovery by measuring and adapting the length and extension of specific muscles or muscle groups.

Stretching has numerous benefits, including some that are beneficial to our minds. There are different types of stretching exercises. Let's look at these five easy and simple stretching exercises for seniors.

What time of day should you stretch?

There isn't a right or wrong moment to stretch. Self-motivation is already a perfect starting point. When you think it's the ideal time for you, take action. Starting as soon as you wake up, stretch. It is beneficial to gently engage your muscles with some stretching after spending the night curled up in bed.

In contrast, don't be surprised; your flexibility won't be at its greatest. Your body has indeed been immobilized for six to nine hours. Perhaps you're stiff. Before beginning your stretching, perform a few joint mobility exercises (pelvic rotation, arm motions, lateral, frontal, anterior leg movements, and cervical mobility).

Additionally, you can do it right before bed to unwind after a long day. You'll definitely nod out! Always avoid stretching shortly after eating. You have a feeling that now is not the greatest time. Keep in mind that stretching requires regularity, much like physical activity.

Create your own pattern.

Ten minutes every day, 20 minutes every other day, or even two 40-minute sessions per week. Everyone needs to discover their own pattern based on their timetable. A stretching session should run for 20 minutes, with each position held for no less than 20 seconds.

What exercises promote flexibility?

There are many physical activities to increase flexibility:

- Ta-chi is a martial art that blends calmness, focus, and self-control. It is based on repeated rotations of the body's center of gravity while bending the legs.
- Yoga, which uses a combination of breathing exercises to move the body gently and tone the muscles deeply, helps reduce stress and increase oxygenation.
- The best exercise for lengthening muscles, tendons, and ligaments is stretching. Aches and muscle contractures are also avoided. Even the feeling of exhaustion can be lessened by it.

Remember that the muscles' ability to stretch and contract quickly declines dramatically without exercise. The tendons may be the site of inflammation or, in severe circumstances, a partial or complete rupture.

How to determine your flexibility

All you have to do to demonstrate your flexibility is:

- Stretch your legs out as you stand up.

- Arm length apart and feet together.

- Lean forward naturally and gradually.

- That's okay if your hands are below your knees!

- To go back to the vertical, remember to bend your legs fully.

Three ways to stretch to improve your flexibility:

1.The "dynamic" stretch: should be used to warm up your body before an activity.

2.Stretching, considered "passive," is done more often after exercise for improved healing, combat pains, and general body relaxation.

3.The "postural" stretches can be used at any time to enhance your appearance, relieve tension, and raise your body's core temperature.

Importance Of Stretching Exercise

1.Stretching eases arthritis and low back pain:

Osteoarthritis and spinal stenosis are prominent causes of lower back discomfort in older persons. The weakening of the cartilage in the joints results in osteoarthritis, the most common kind of arthritis in the joints effects in osteoarthritis, the most common type of arthritis. Usually, the accompanying low back discomfort is intermittent. In addition to osteoarthritis of the low back, arthritis commonly manifests in the neck, fingers, toes, hips, and knees.

Narrowing of the bone channel used by the spinal nerves or cord is known as spinal stenosis. Sciatica symptoms include tingling, weakness, and numbness in the low back, buttocks, and legs due to compression of the spinal nerves. While osteoarthritis and spinal stenosis are both inevitable aging conditions and cannot be prevented, the pain they cause can be controlled with stretching exercises. Seniors benefit from regular stretching by increasing their range of motion, suppleness, and flexibility to reduce stiffness in the affected joints. Understandably, stretching or moving these joints may be uncomfortable and challenging.

It is suggested to warm up tense muscles with a heat pack before stretching and, in the opposite direction, to cool down muscles with an ice pack after.

2.Stretching can help with poor posture.

Our body's connective tissue, including ligaments and tendons, loses water as we age, making it less elastic and flexible. Poor posture develops over time due to the chest and shoulder's ligaments and tendons becoming tighter and due to years spent slouching at a desk. – Forward head position, rounded shoulders and upper back, and forward-pressing hips are all signs of poor posture. Our spine's organic S-curve compresses. This could cause pain in the lower back, between the shoulder blades, etc. Consistent stretching is a simple way to increase flexibility. You will have more range of motion due to this helping to loosen tight ligaments, tendons, and muscles. Supplementing seniors strength training is also a good idea.

3.Stretching boosts energy and blood flow.

Using movement to stretch your muscles, dynamic stretching is a low-intensity technique of stretching versus static stretching, which involves stretching when your body is still.

Dynamic stretches will lengthen your muscles as well as improve blood flow and nutrient distribution throughout the body. Increasing the body's energy levels as a result. Increased vitality is crucial for older persons to keep their independence, stay connected to their social networks, and age healthily overall.

4.Stress in the mind and body is released

5.Increases muscle tone and reduces some injury risks (strains, tears, tendinitis, etc.)

6.It makes the nervous and hormonal systems function better

7.Relieves joints and tendons and efficiently combats stress

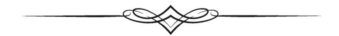

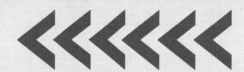

FIFTY STRETCHING EXERCISES FOR SENIORS

PART 1

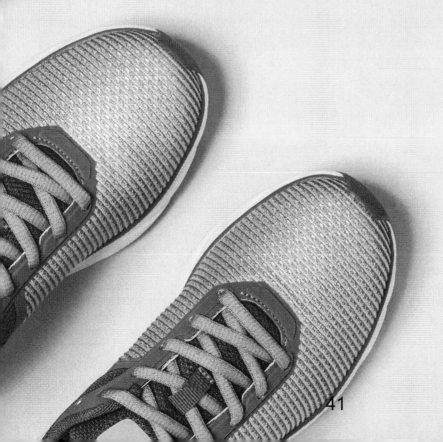

STRETCHING EXERCISE FOR ARMS

Easy Exercises

1-STRETCH WRISTS

- Straighten out your right arm in front of you at shoulder height, palm upward.
- Press the palm and fingers of your right hand toward the ground using your opposite hand.
- Hold for 5 seconds, then restart where you left off. It's one rep, then.
- Do three repetitions on both the right and left sides.

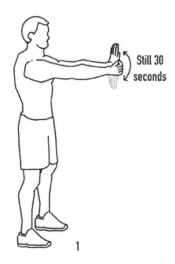

2 - CROSS BODY STRETCH

- Cross your right arm at shoulder height to the left side after extending it straight in front of your body.
- With your left arm, push your right upper arm toward your left shoulder.
- Hold for 30 seconds, then restart where you left off. It's one rep, then.
- Do three repetitions on both the right and left sides.

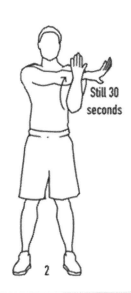

3 - TRICEPS STRETCH

- Straighten your right arm overhead such that the top of it is adjacent to your ear.
- Reach your fingertips near your shoulder blades while bending your right elbow. With your left hand, gently draw your right elbow inside to help with the stretch.
- Hold for 30 seconds, then restart where you left off. It's one rep, then.
- Do three repetitions on both the right and left sides.

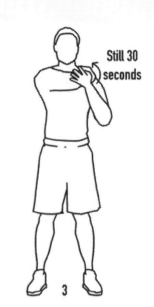

4 - LONG ARM STRETCHES

- Breathe as you gently start to spread your arms as far apart as you can safely do so.
- Feel the stretch over your arms and chest, and your hands should be facing forward.
- Breathe out as you return to the beginning position by pushing your arms together.

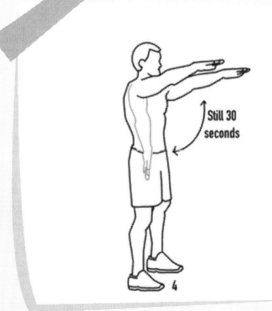

5 - SHOULDER STRETCH

You can open up your shoulder joint and reduce muscle pain and degeneration by performing this straightforward shoulder stretch.

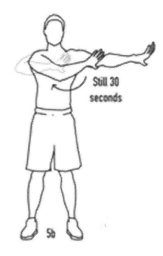

- As tall as you can, stand or sit.
- With your opposite hand, grab one of your arms and slowly, delicately drag it across your chest until you begin to feel a stretch in your shoulder. (Be sure to maintain your elbow below shoulder height while stretching.)
- Hold this posture for ten to thirty seconds, then switch to the opposite arm.

For your stretching exercises to be as effective as possible, you can perform this stretch while standing or sitting, depending on your preference.

6 - OVERHEAD SIDE STRETCH

An excellent and simple exercise to relax your stomach, back, and shoulders is the overhead side stretch, also known as the standing side stretch.

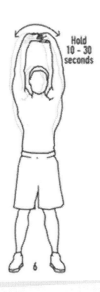

- Extend your arms over your head while standing with your feet shoulder-width apart, interlocking your fingers if you like.
- Leaning slightly to the left while maintaining a long torso. Return to the center after holding this position for 10 to 30 seconds;
- On the right side, carry out the same stretch.

7 - ARM CIRCLE

- As you slowly raise your arms until they are stretched forth
- Breathe as you move your arms in broad, circular motions in the air.
- It is advisable that you begin gently and steadily, picking up speed as you become more at ease. Your muscles will have more time to adapt and participate in the stretch.
- After finishing this in one direction, switch it up and rotate your arms the other way, for example. If you move your arms clockwise, switch to moving them counterclockwise.

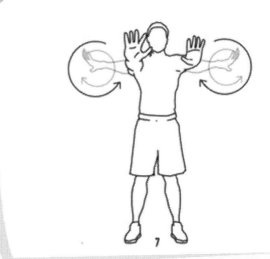

8 - WALL BICEP STRETCH

- Take a deep breath and firmly place your palm against the wall to secure yourself before beginning this stretch.
- otate your body away from the wall gradually.
- s you fully commit to the stretch, breathe.
- You should feel a stretch in your arm and shoulder muscles as you perform this upper arm stretch.

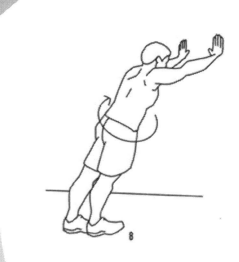

9 - SHOULDER STRETCH

You can open up your shoulder joint and reduce muscle pain and degeneration by performing this straightforward shoulder stretch.

As tall as you can, stand or sit.
- With your opposite hand, grab one of your arms and slowly, delicately drag it across your chest until you begin to feel a stretch in your shoulder. (Be sure to maintain your elbow below shoulder height while stretching.)
- Hold this posture for ten to thirty seconds, then switch to the opposite arm.
- For your stretching exercises to be as effective as possible, you can perform this stretch while standing or sitting, depending on your preference.

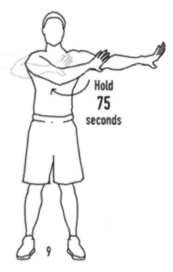

10 - OVERHEAD SIDE STRETCH

An excellent and simple exercise to relax your stomach, back, and shoulders is the overhead side stretch, also known as the standing side stretch.

- Extend your arms over your head while standing with your feet shoulder-width apart, interlocking your fingers if you like.
- Leaning slightly to the left while maintaining a long torso. Return to the center after holding this position for 10 to 30 seconds;
- On the right side, carry out the same stretch.
- You can perform this exercise while seated is another fantastic feature.

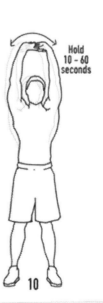

11 - HAND FLEXION AND STRETCH

- Sit or stand tall, to begin with. One arm should be extended in front of you at or just below shoulder height.
- Press down on the top of your extended hand with the opposite hand while keeping your extended arm straight.
- Until you feel a stretch on the top of your forearm and wrist, slowly bend your wrist downward so that your fingertips point toward the floor.
- Continue on the opposite side after holding for at least 30 seconds.

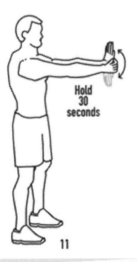

12 - THREAD THE NEEDLE

- On all fours, place your hands below your shoulders and your knees squarely beneath your hips.
- With your palm facing up, raise your right hand and carefully cross it across to the left.
- Place your right shoulder under your torso and tilt your head to the left.
- Be careful not to sag onto your shoulder.
- For 30 seconds, maintain this posture.
- Release gradually, then return to your starting position.
- On the other side, repeat.

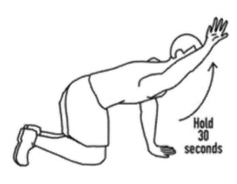

48

STRETCHING EXERCISE
FOR THE NECK

13 - NECK STRETCH

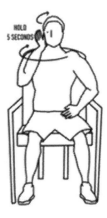

- Sit down in a chair. Roll your shoulders back and look ahead, keeping both of your feet firmly on the ground.
- Grasp your left thigh with your left hand. Hold onto the chair's seat as an alternative.
- Your right hand should be used to cup the right side of your head. The starting place is here.
- To lengthen your neck, bend it to the right and softly press with your right hand.
- Avoid tilting your head or tucking your chin. Keep your neck straight.
- For 30 seconds, keep the stretch in place.
- Switch sides and relax.
- Follow this five times.

13

14 - SIDE BEND STRETCH

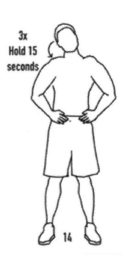

- Try to touch your ear to your shoulder by tilting your head to one side.
- For 15 seconds, maintain the posture.
- From the position, unwind.
- Three times on each side, repeat.

14

15 - STRAIGHT-NECK STRETCH

- Slowly gaze down as though inspecting a hand or pocket after slightly turning the head to one side.
- For 15 seconds, maintain the posture.
- From the position, unwind.
- Three times on each side, repeat.

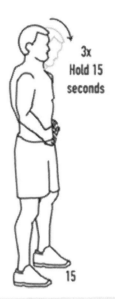

16 - NECK TURN

- Keep your chin level and only go as far as is comfortable while you turn your head to one side.
- Hold a mild tension in your neck muscles for five seconds.
- Repeat on the other side after bringing your head back to the center.
- Repeat five times on each side.

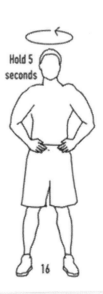

17 - NECK EXTENSION STRETCH

- Keep your shoulders down and back while sitting up straight in your chair.
- As far back as you feel comfortable while staring up at the ceiling, tilt your head straight back.
- Never try to push through discomfort.
- Hold for the allotted amount of time.

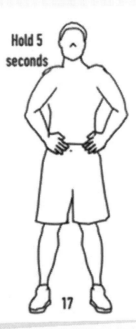

18 - NECK SIDE FLEXION STRETCH

- Keep your shoulders down and back while sitting up straight in your chair.
- Your ear should be at shoulder level.
- Keep your shoulder relaxed and avoid raising it to your ear.
- Go as far as you are at ease with.
- Affix a hand to the side of your head and gently press down to lengthen the stretch.
- Hold for the allotted time, then switch sides.

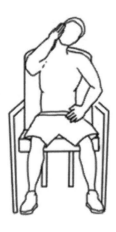

19 - NECK FLEXION STRETCH

- Keep your shoulders down and back while sitting up straight in your chair.
- As far as it seems comfortable, lower your chin toward your chest. Back of neck stretch is what you'll experience.
- Affix your hands on the back of your head and gently press down to lengthen the stretch.
- Hold for the given period of time.

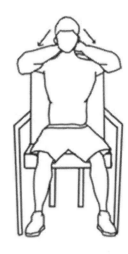

19

20 - LEVATOR SCAPULAR STRETCH

- Keep your shoulders down and back while sitting up straight in your chair.
- To stabilize your shoulder blade, place the hand on the side you are stretching behind your shoulder. If you cannot do this, carry out the exercise without putting one hand behind your shoulder.
- Turn your head to one side at about a 45-degree angle, then lower it as if you were gazing at your knee on that side. You will feel a stretch when you glance behind the neck and shoulder on the opposite side. (This muscle is referred to as the Levator Scapular.)
- Place your palm on the back of your head and gently press down to lengthen the stretch.
- Hold for the designated time, then repeat on the other side.

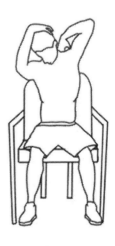

20

53

Difficult Exercises

21 - NECK ISOMETRICS

- Your forehead should be touched without allowing your hand to move. Push your head against it. Take a 5-second hold.
- Push with your palm while placing it on the back of your head. Take a 5-second hold.
- Push with your hand while placing it on your head's right side. Take a 5-second hold.
- Put your left hand on your head's left side and press. Take a 5-second hold.
- This easy strengthening exercise should be repeated 3–5 times.

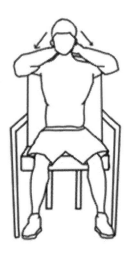

19

22 - HEAD LIFTS

- Place your feet must be on the floor, your knees bent, and your arms by your sides.
- Stabilize your spine by contracting your core.
- Your chin should travel toward your chest as you lift your head off the floor. When you reach the top, pause before going back to the beginning.
- Keep your shoulders flat on the ground as you carry out this neck-strengthening exercise.

Perform this ten to fifteen times.

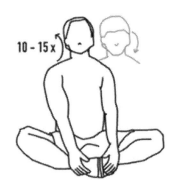

10 - 15 x

22

23 - WALL ANGELS

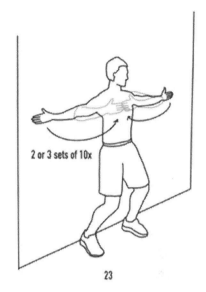

- Place your back against a wall as you stand.
- Steps: forward with slightly bowed knees and your feet shoulder-width apart.
- Make a "T" formation with your arms raised out to the sides. Your hands, elbows, and backs of your forearms should be against the wall.
- Your elbows should be bent at a 90-degree angle to resemble a goalpost in football.
- Your left and right hands' fingertips should touch when you spread your arms in front of you. At all times, keep your back and elbows up against the wall.
- Return your arms to the position at the goalposts.

Practice two or three sets of ten repetitions each.

24 - PRONE COBRA

- Put a hand towel that has been rolled up on the forehead while lying face down for comfort.
- Put the arms at your sides with the palms facing the ground.
- Put the tongue on the mouth's roof (this aids in balancing and strengthening the muscles in the front of the neck).
- Lift your hands off the ground while pinching your shoulder blades together.
- Thumbs up, palms out, and elbows rolled in.
- Lift the forehead gently off the towel while maintaining a straight line of vision for the ground (do not tip the head back and look forward).
- For ten seconds, maintain the position.
- Make ten repetitions.

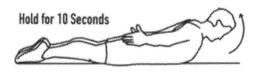

STRETCHING EXERCISES FOR THE CHEST

25 - PARALLEL BAR DIPS

- Position your arms on parallel bars in front of you while you stand.
- Hold out your hands at shoulder distance.
- Bend your waist and lower your body until your forearms are within an inch of being parallel with the floor while keeping your feet slightly wider than hip-width apart.
- After a brief pause, press up for 8–12 repetitions in each set.

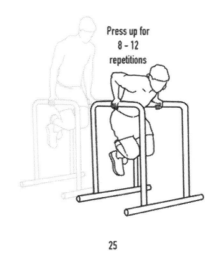

26 - CABLE CHEST FLY'S

- Grip the cable handles while standing with your back to the cable machine. Leaning forward slightly, put one foot in front of the other.
- Maintain a straight back. Pull the handlebars in front of your chest toward one another until your hand's contact, keeping your arms slightly bent.
- Then, gradually let go so that both arms can regain their initial positions simultaneously.
- Throughout the entire workout, keep your core engaged.

Change the position of your feet after 10 to 15 repetitions and carry out the exercise once more for a second set.

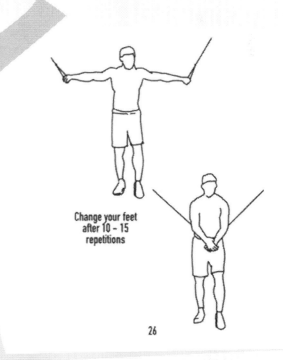

27 - TRADITIONAL PUSH-UPS

- Start by getting down on your knees, with your legs a few inches apart and your hands a little wider than your shoulders.
- Put yourself in a high plank position by extending your arms and legs such that your knees are off the ground.
- Keep your head, neck, shoulders, back, and knees straight as you gradually lower your body until your chest is only a few inches above the ground.
- Come back to the starting position by pushing with your arms and chest.
- For two or three sets, repeat this motion eight to ten times.

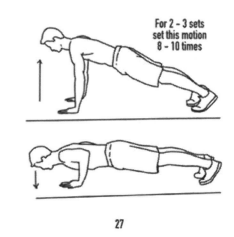

For 2 - 3 sets set this motion 8 - 10 times

27

28 - SCAPULAR PUSH-UPS

- Start in a high plank posture for this push-up variation, keeping your feet a few inches apart and your hands shoulder-width apart.
- Squeeze your shoulder blades slowly toward one another while maintaining a straight back and arms, and then let go.
- The body should minimally move up and down less than during a regular push-up.
- Perform three sets of eight scapular push-ups.

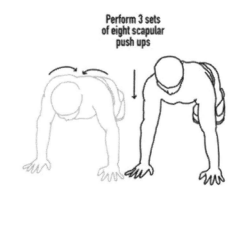

Perform 3 sets of eight scapular push ups

28

29 - CHEST STRETCH

- Lie down comfortably on the bed or sit on a chair.
- Take hold of a resistance or therapeutic band; likewise, put your arms out in front of you, keeping them shoulder-width apart. This is where everything begins.
- Stretch your chest muscles by spreading your arms widely.
- Return to the starting position after holding the position for 5 seconds. Through each stage, maintain a normal breathing pattern.
- Perform this ten to fifteen times.

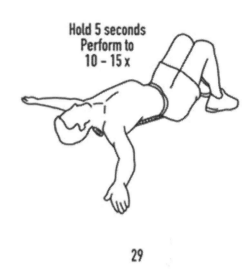

Hold 5 seconds
Perform to
10 – 15 x

29

STRETCHING EXERCISES FOR LEGS

Easy Exercises

30 - ANKLE CIRCLES

- Place yourself erect in a chair.
- Place your left foot firmly on the ground. Draw a circle with your right foot while lifting your right knee into the air. Twenty times.
- With your right foot, step in the opposite direction of the circle. Twenty times total.
- Use your left foot to carry out the same exercise.
-

Try stretching your knee out if you cannot lift it into the air. For a greater challenge, try performing the workout while standing. Standing ankle circles will test you and help you gain better balance.

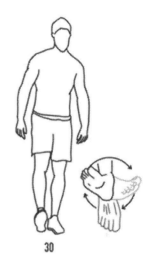

30

31 - KNEE EXTENSION

- Lie down on the floor with your feet up in a chair.
- Take a deep breath as you slowly lift and straighten your left knee in front of you. As much as you can, tuck your toes in toward you. Hold for a short while.
- As you carefully lower your left foot to the ground, exhale. Repeat ten times.
- Do the same with your right knee.

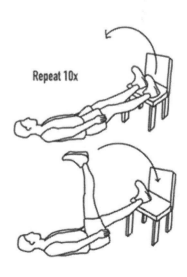

Repeat 10x

31

61

32 - CALF RAISES

- Holding onto the chair's back will help you balance while you stand behind it. Maintain a straight back.
- Take a breath and slowly raise yourself to your toes or as high as feels comfortable for you. Avoid moving the rest of your body.
- Breathe out as you slowly descend to the floor with your feet flat.
- Ten times in total.
- Try it without holding on to the chair for added difficulty. Alternatively, try using fewer fingers.

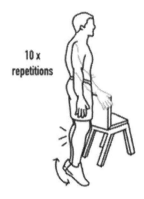

10 x repetitions

32

33 - MARCHING HIP

- Lie down on the floor with your feet up in a chair.
- As you carefully raise your left knee as high as possible, take a breath.
- Breathe out as you slowly descend to the ground. Repeat ten times in total.
- Do the same with your right knee.

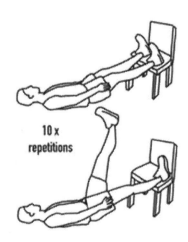

10 x repetitions

33

34 - STANDING KNEE FLEXION

- Before beginning this workout, briefly stretch your hamstring.
- Holding onto the chair's back for support, stand up straight.
- Inhale as you raise your left foot slowly behind you while bending your left knee. As far as you can comfortably manage, try to bend your knee to a right angle. Don't sag your hips.
- Breathe as you slowly bring your left foot back to a flat position on the ground.
- Ten times in total.
- Similarly, step with your right foot.
-

Try it without holding on to the chair for added difficulty. Alternatively, try using fewer fingers.

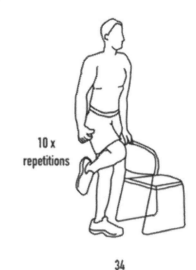

10 x repetitions

34

35 - SIDE HIP RAISE

- Holding onto the chair's back for balance, stand up straight behind it with your ribcage raised. Hip distance should separate your feet.
- As you raise your left leg to the side slowly, inhale. Maintain a straight angle with your foot and point your toes forward. Go up as high as you feel comfortable. Avoid bending at the hips.
- As you carefully lower your leg to the ground, exhale.
- Ten times in total.
- Apply the same technique to your other leg.
- Try it without holding on to the chair for added difficulty. Alternatively, try using fewer fingers.

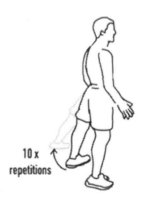

10 x repetitions

35

63

36 - HEEL STAND

- Holding onto the chair's back for balance, stand up straight behind it with your ribcage raised.
- Breathe as you slowly bounce back onto your heels while erecting your toes.
- Breathe in as you slowly return your toes to the earth.
- Ten times in total.
- Holding onto the chair's back for balance, stand up straight behind it with your ribcage raised.

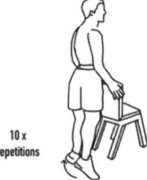

10 x
repetitions

36

37 - SIT TO STAND

- With your knees resting on the chair's seat, take a tall stance in front of it.
- Breathe in as you slowly lean forward and budge your hips toward the direction of the chair. Before you sit down, pause.
- Exhale after a little pause as you steadily bring your body back to standing.
- Repeat ten times.

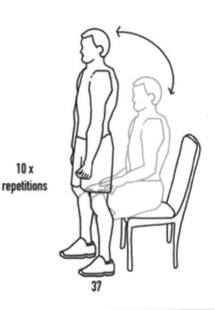

10 x
repetitions

37

Difficult Exercises

38 - STRAIGHT LEG RAISE

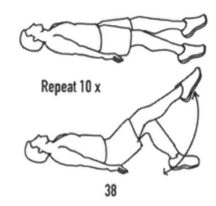

Repeat 10 x

38

- Lie flat on your back. Ensure that the floor contacts the lower part of your back. Your right leg should remain straight as you begin with your left knee bent and your left foot on the ground. Maintain flat palms on the floor.
- Take a deep breath as you slowly raise your right leg, keeping it straight to the level of your left knee. Hold the position for some seconds (10) if you can.
- As you put your right leg back in the beginning position, exhale.
- Repeat ten times.

Likewise, perform with you left leg.

39 - PARTIAL SQUATS

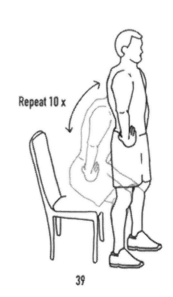

Repeat 10 x

39

- In front of a chair, stand straight up. Hold onto the back of it for balance while maintaining your high ribcage and shoulder blades. Inhale.
- As you slowly bend your knees as far as you can without discomfort, exhale. Keep your upper body straight at all times.
- As you gently revert to the starting position, take a breath.
- Repeat ten times.
- Try it without holding on to the chair for added difficulty. Alternatively, try using fewer fingers.

40 - HIP EXTENSION

- Holding onto the chair's back for balance, stand up straight behind it with your ribcage raised.
- Breathe as you progressively extend your left foot back while maintaining a straight knee. Keep your foot at a straight angle.
- As you carefully reposition your left foot to the beginning position, let out a breath.
- Repeat ten times.
- Then, switch sides and use your right foot to repeat the action.

Try it without holding on to the chair for added difficulty. Alternatively, try using fewer fingers.

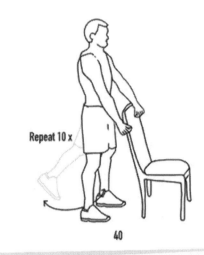

Repeat 10 x

40

41 - STEP-UPS

- At the bottom of the stairs, raise your body straight. For stability, cling to the railing.
- Steps: up slowly, placing your right foot firmly and completely on the step.
- Use your left foot to follow.
- Steps: back down slowly, first with your right foot and then your left.
- Repeat ten times.
- Start by pushing up with your left foot instead of your right.

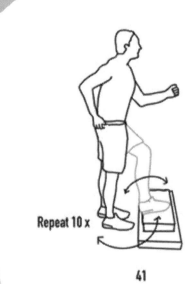

Repeat 10 x

41

42 - STANDING HIP FLEXOR

This stretch, one of many hip flexor exercises for seniors, is excellent for releasing tightness or soreness in your hips. Remember that this is a challenging exercise and might be more appropriate for people with greater experience.

- Grab a sturdy chair, then stand with your feet facing the back of it. Make sure you are far enough away from the chair so that you can pull your leg up.
- Then, while still holding on to the chair with both hands, lift the opposite leg toward your chest while bending the knee and bringing it as close to your chest as you can.
- Repeat holding this posture for 10 to 15 seconds.

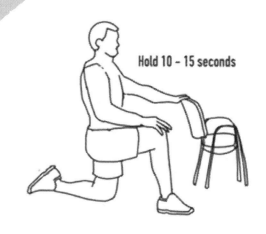

Hold 10 - 15 seconds

42

43 - TOE LIFTS

Seniors who perform this leg-strengthening exercise also benefit from improved balance.

- Straighten your body, extend your arms in front of you, and stand on your toes as tall as possible.
- Then gradually lower yourself. You should raise and lower yourself around 15 times.

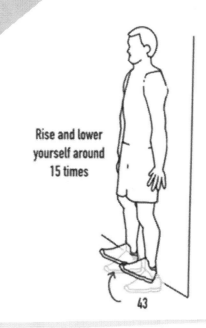

Rise and lower yourself around 15 times

43

44 - REVERSE LUNGE

- With both hands on the chair, stand tall.
- Just before the floor, take a big stride backward in the opposite direction.
- Return to your feet and repeat with the other leg.
- Throughout the workout, maintain your upright posture and watch that your front foot's knee does not extend over the line of your toes.
- For each set of repetitions, repeat.

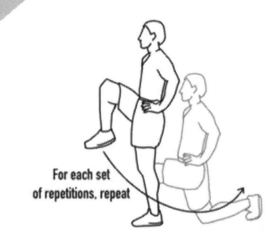

For each set
of repetitions, repeat

44

45 - HIP ABSTRACTS (LEG SIDEWAYS - STRAIGHT)

- Hold on to your chair while standing erect and keeping your feet close together.
- Bring your foot back together smoothly after bringing your leg out to the side.
- During this exercise, make sure your toes are pointed forward. You should also avoid leaning or hunching your pelvis.
- Change legs after each repeat to complete the set.

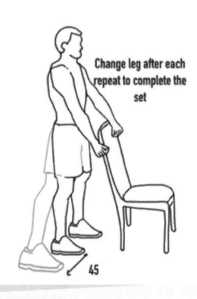

Change leg after each
repeat to complete the
set

45

46 - SEATED KNEE EXTENSIONS

- Keep your shoulders back and down when sitting tall.
- Extend one knee while raising one leg.
- Before lowering your leg back down, hold the position at the top of the exercise for a brief moment while contracting the muscles in front of your thigh.
- Make careful to move slowly and deliberately.
- Alternate legs and extend them fully (leg completely straight).
- Repeat for the set repetitions.

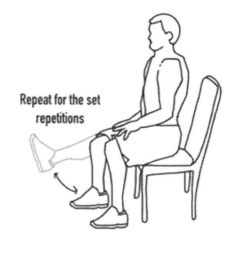

Repeat for the set repetitions

46

47 - HIP ADDUCTIONS (THIGH SQUEEZES)

- Shuffle forward to the center of the chair while sitting tall.
- Put the object between your knees while in this posture by utilizing a cushion or a towel that has been rolled up.
- Make sure your knees align with your feet as you bring them in.
- You will now lightly squeeze the cushion with your knees while holding it in place.
- Relax after five seconds of holding this.
- Repeat for the set repetitions.

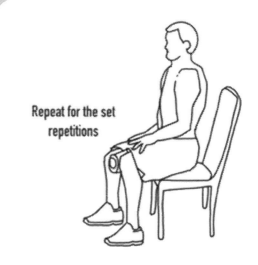

Repeat for the set repetitions

47

48 - SQUAT

- Place your feet shoulder-width apart while standing tall.
- Keep both hands firmly in the chair.
- Take a chair-like position by leaning back and hinging at the hips.
- ØSit back no more than 90 degrees before standing back up.
- Put the same amount of weight on both legs.
- Throughout the workout, ensure your knees don't cross your toes' lines and aren't sliding inward.
- Repeat for the set repetitions.

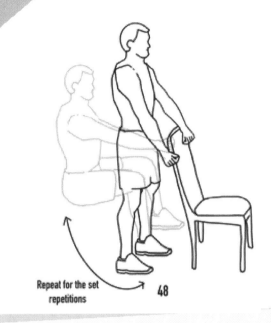

Repeat for the set repetitions

48

49 - LUNGES

Lunges are a wonderful exercise for your hips and quadriceps. Place your hands on your hips, stand up straight, and maintain a shoulder-width distance between your feet.

- Steps: forward with one foot as you exhale, keeping your torso straight and the other foot firmly planted on the ground.
- As you get back to where you were, take a breath.
- Repeat the exercise while switching the legs.

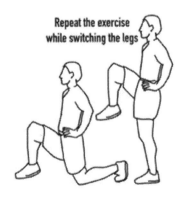

Repeat the exercise while switching the legs

49

70

50 - STEPS-UPS

Your quads and glutes will get stronger, and this exercise will make climbing stairs easier.

- Holding onto the railing will provide stability and support when you stand at the foot of the stairs or a few steps up.
- Place one foot firmly on the step in front of you as you rise, then use the other to complete the ascent of the one step.
- To get back to your starting position, take a step back with your first foot and then your second.

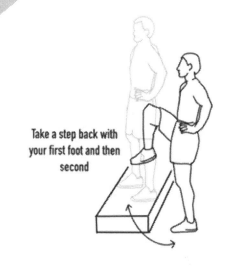

Take a step back with your first foot and then second

50

BOOK 2: BALANCE EXERCISES FOR SENIORS

What is a balance exercise?

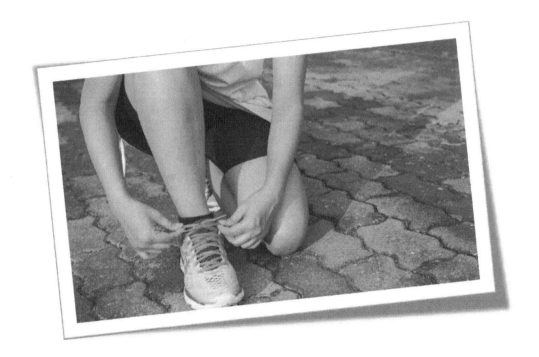

Balance exercises help you gain more control and stability over your body's position. Exercises that improve balance are especially crucial for older adults because as you age, proprioception, the sense of where you are in space, deteriorates and makes it harder to maintain balance. Exercises for balance training include strengthening your legs and core, two muscles important for maintaining your balance. These exercises can increase stability and assist in preventing falls. Fall risk is extremely significant for older people when dealing with issues that limit their movement.

They experience it due to their general loss of muscle mass and the resulting joint pain, gradually weakening them. They may experience a decline in cognitive abilities due to other age-related illnesses. A number of elements can lead to falls in seniors that have major repercussions (e.g., falling down the stairs). Through seniors balance exercises, balance and muscle strength can be improved, two crucial components to reducing the risk of falling. This is a valuable asset for seniors mobility security and accident prevention. Seniors can accomplish this by exercising daily at home quite easily or by participating in sports or jogging.

Numerous problems that older adults deal with can limit their movement. Most people experience joint discomfort from arthritis as they age, and muscle mass generally declines. Dizziness, weakness, and changes in cognitive abilities can also be brought on by age-related disorders like Alzheimer's disease, Parkinson's disease, osteoporosis, vision loss, and heart disease (as well as the prescription medications used to treat them). Even if they are small in number, the combination of these factors significantly raises an older person's risk of falling.

Many older people and their caretakers worry a lot about the possibility of a fall inflicting injuries, and for a good reason. An older person's risk of falling increases by half, along with their chance of dying sooner. More than 95% of hip fractures are caused by falls, which can have a terrible and frequently permanent impact on a senior's physical and mental health.

Fortunately, consistent practice of balance exercises helps to enhance balance and lower the danger of falling, as does combining them with muscle-strengthening activities or gentle gym. The most crucial thing is to practice consistently. To ensure their mobility and avoid accidents, elders might do these activities while being accompanied. As a result, one of the most crucial things you can do to prevent this kind of dramatic incident is to learn how to maintain equilibrium. Exercises that improve balance should be done regularly by all elders. Seniors balance exercises reduce the risk of injury by 61% in the case of a fall for seniors who consistently perform them. Regularly doing balance exercises for seniors helps to build stronger bones and muscle tissue.

The following are some fall risks:

- Weakness.

- Poor balance

- Polypharmacy: using more than three medications

- Sedentary kind of life

- Health issues

- Cognitive impairments, etc.

Importance of Balance Exercises

1.Increasing muscular strength

Your muscles can swiftly produce more power due to muscle strengthening through balance. You'll be able to sprint faster and jump higher if they have more force to work with. Practically every discipline, such as boxing, that calls for quick, powerful movements can benefit from balance, which also helps develop overall functional strength.

2.Preventing falls

You can manage your core and limbs more deftly by using balance exercises. This not only helps you walk more gracefully, but it also keeps you from falling. When you have good balance, you may modify your body posture more quickly and respond swiftly to unanticipated changes in height or unseen hazards.

Not only can avoiding falls help you prevent bodily harm like broken hips, but it also gives you more confidence. When you have a good balance, you can leave the house without worrying about falling every time. Even if you're young, having this subconscious understanding gives you more self-assurance among other people and in social situations. When your balancing system is functioning at its best, you can respond to slips more rapidly, decreasing the likelihood that you'll fall.

3.Reversing Age-Related Balance Loss

Our capacity for balance lessens as we age. For instance, the amount of time a person can stand on one leg is a crucial indicator of lifespan. Balance is a complicated combination of brain, muscle, and inner ear functions.

The coordination between these three systems degrades with time if you don't train and maintain balance, making it more difficult to stand up straight and maintain good posture.

However, the practice maintains everything functioning as if your body were much younger, assisting you in avoiding some of the balance problems that could come with aging.

4.Strengthen Joint Stability

The joints in your ankles, knees, hips, and shoulders all become stronger when you balance. Your joints are less likely to sustain injuries when they are stable. Acute pain to more serious sprains and breaks are all possible with joint injuries. Ankle and knee pain are common among seniors. By including balancing exercises in your daily regimen, you can keep your joints stable and decrease the likelihood of injury.

5.Improve Your Posture

You may quickly improve your posture by focusing on your balance for just a few minutes each day.

Your body will need to adapt to its natural form as you balance using static and dynamic positions. Additionally, by strengthening your legs, back, core, and buttocks, you'll automatically be able to stand (or sit) up straighter.

6.Prevent Back Pain

It's not uncommon for people to experience lower back pain, especially as they age. Weak abdominal muscles, which serve as the spine's front attachment point, are frequently to blame for this. Your back will have to work more to keep you upright if they're weak.

Your core muscles will naturally get stronger if you incorporate balance exercises into your daily routine. You may stand, sit, and move about pain-free by pulling your weight via your abdominal muscles, relieving strain on your lower back.

7.Enhance Cognitive Performance

Being balanced requires a lot of mental effort! You don't think about it often, but after concentrating on standing on one foot for a while or attempting to balance on a moving surface, you'll realize that you need to focus merely to maintain your balance. Your general health will benefit from all of this mental effort.

According to studies, seniors who consistently do balance exercises can more efficiently improve their memory and spatial awareness than healthy persons who concentrate on cardiac workouts.

8.Higher Agility

The practice of balancing also has another benefit. Your agile movements will improve with training. Your ability to maneuver with control will be enhanced by having excellent agility.

Fewer falls occur when a body is more agile. You'll be better positioned to prevent slips and other incidents that could result in serious injury. Your ability to hold your ground will be improved if you have better balance in a fixed position.

9.Increased Strength

Other benefits of balancing training include increased strength. You are not required to lift heavy iron for the rest of your life. Your nervous system will be instructed to build up your muscles if your balance improves. Small stabilizer muscles are triggered by balance training. You can become stronger by working your muscles. Your stabilizer muscles will contract to keep you balanced if you don't have adequate bodily balance. Your larger muscles also have to work harder to keep you steady.

Your neural system will connect with the muscles as your balance training plan progresses, giving you the strength you need to perform more strenuous physical activities.

10.Improves Long Term Health

Adding balance exercises to your everyday activity is the ideal challenge. It inspires you to continue making improvements to your long-term health. Your balance declines as you become older. You must balance your training to stay healthy and avoid fractures and falls.

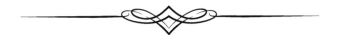

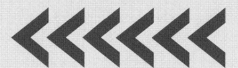

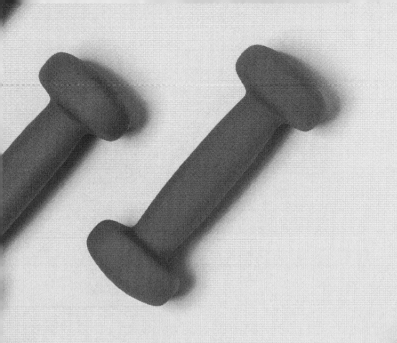

FIFTY
BALANCE
EXERCISES
FOR SENIORS

PART 2

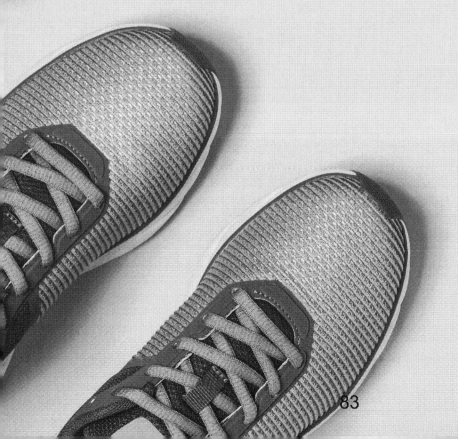

Easy Exercises

1 - HEEL-TOE WALKING

- Stand up and place your right foot just in front of your left foot: the heel of the right foot touches the tip of the toes of the left foot.
- Move the left foot in front of the right foot (putting your weight on the heel).
- Put weight on your toes.

Repeat this exercise 20 times (which equates to 20 steps).

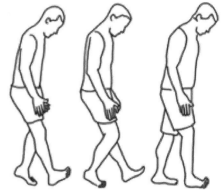

Repeat this exercise 20 times (which equates to 20 steps).

1

2 - THE PINK FLAMINGO

- While standing on one foot, place the arch of the other foot, slightly to the side, against the calf of the rigid leg.
- Regain support by putting your foot back after roughly ten seconds of balance maintenance.

- For each foot, perform this exercise five more times.

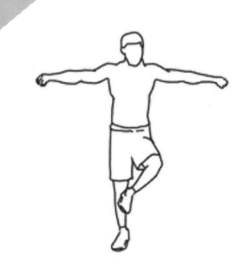

Hold 5 seconds

3 - MAKE CIRCLES

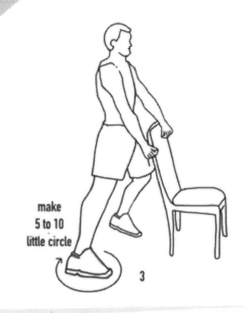

- Use a chair to assist yourself while carrying out this exercise.
- Extend your right leg laterally while slightly bending the knee of your left leg.
- With the tip of the right foot, make 5 to 10 little circles on the pelvis with both hands without letting it touch the ground.

make
5 to 10
little circle

3

4 - HEAD ROTATIONS

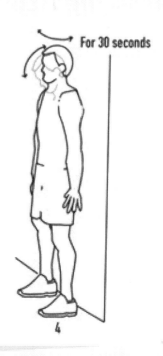

For 30 seconds

- Place your feet a little apart and stand straight up, level with the breadth of your hips (do not hesitate to lean on a piece of furniture or a wall).
- or 30 seconds, move your head up Fand down and side to side while remaining motionless.
-

If you become lightheaded throughout the exercise, stop for a few seconds and then resume it by moving your head more slowly (do not continue the exercise if the dizziness persists).

4

5 - STANCE ON ONE LEG

- Hold on to the back of a strong, stationary chair (not one with wheels).
- Balance on your left foot while raising your right foot.
- As long as you can, maintain this posture, then alternate legs.

The objective is to maintain this position for a minute while standing on one foot without clinging to the chair.

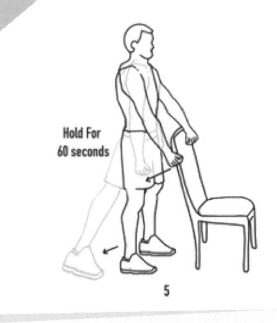

Hold For
60 seconds

5

6 - REAR LEG RAISE

- Steps: back from a chair.
- Slowly raise your right leg back without bending your knees or pointing your toes.
- After a few periods of holding, slowly lower your leg.
- For each leg, repeat 10 to 15 times.

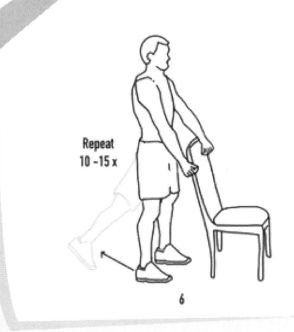

Repeat
10 -15 x

6

7 - STANCE ON ONE LEG WITH ARMS

- Your feet should be together when you stand next to a chair with your arms at your sides. Put your left hand in the air above your head.
- After then, slowly raise your left foot off the ground.
- Maintain this posture for ten seconds.

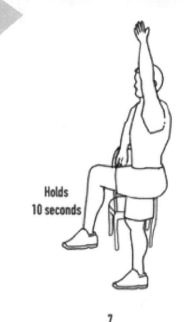

Holds
10 seconds

7

8 - LATERAL LEG RAISE

- Put your feet slightly apart and take a position behind the chair.
- Lift your right leg gradually to the side.
- Maintain a straight back, forward-facing toes, and a forward-looking gaze. Gently stoop your right leg.

For each leg, repeat 10 to 15 times.

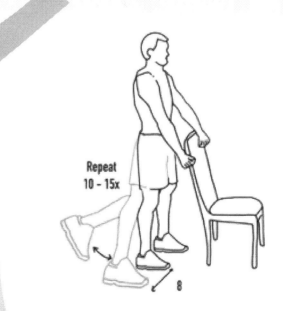

Repeat
10 - 15x

8

9 - BALANCE STICK

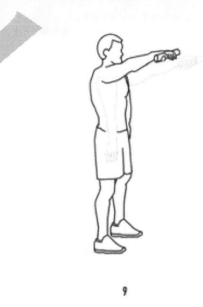

- Hold the stick firmly in your hand, flat on the palm.
- Maintaining the stick straight for as long as possible is the objective of this workout.

To practice your balance on both sides of your body, switch hands.

10 - PUSH-UPS ON THE WALL

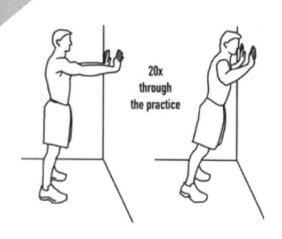

20x
through
the practice

- Place your arm's length in front of a blank wall that isn't covered in artwork, ornaments, windows, or doors.
- Put your palms flat on the wall, shoulder height apart, while leaning slightly forward.
- Maintain a strong ground position with your feet as you progressively get closer to the wall.
- Pull back gently until your arms are straight.

Twenty times through the practice.

11 - MILITARY MARCH IN PLACE

Exercise in front of a counter if you need to hold onto something.

- Raise the right knee as high as you can while standing.
- Lift the left leg first, then lower it.

Raise and lower your legs 20 times.

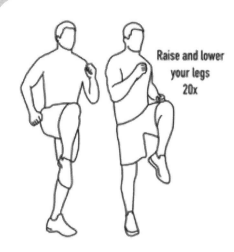

Raise and lower your legs 20x

11

12 - TOE RAISES

- You'll require a seat or a counter.
- Straighten your spine and extend your arms in front of you.
- Stand up on your toes as high as you can, then slowly bring yourself back down. Avoid slouching too much forward on the counter or chair.

Raise and lower yourself 20 times.

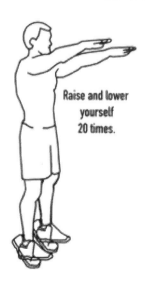

Raise and lower yourself 20 times.

12

13 - SHOULDER ROLLS

- Either standing or sitting is acceptable.
- Roll your shoulders back and down after a gentle ascent to the ceiling.
- Roll them down after doing the same, then forward.

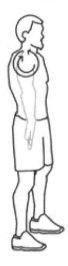

13

14 - ROCK THE BOAT

- Place your feet hip-width apart as you stand.
- As you raise your arms, spread them wide.
- Bring your left heel toward your bottom by raising your left foot off the ground and bending your left knee.
- Maintain this posture for 30 seconds.
- Proceed with the other side, three times on each side.

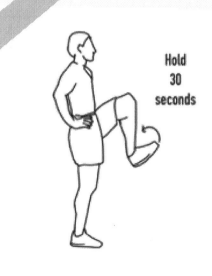

Hold
30
seconds

14

15 - WEIGHT CHANGES

- Place your feet hip-width apart as you stand.
- Place your right foot underweight.
- Your left foot is up.
- For up to 30 seconds, maintain this posture.
- Do the other side next.

Do each side three times.

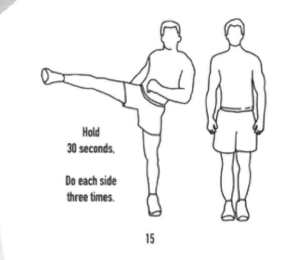

Hold
30 seconds.

Do each side
three times.

15

16 - WALK A TIGHTROPE

- Open wide as you raise your arms.
- Keep your eyes on a fixed point in the distance and proceed straight ahead.
- Hold your foot in place every time you lift it for two to three seconds before stopping.
- Count to 20 or 30 steps.

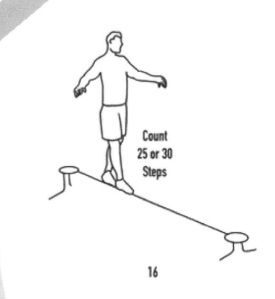

Count
25 or 30
Steps

16

17 - BACK LEG RAISES

- Put your hands on a chair back or a wall.
- Place your right foot underweight.
- Extend your left leg as high as possible while slowly repositioning it.
- For five seconds, maintain this posture.
- Go back to the beginning place.
- Repeat ten times.
- Do the other side next.

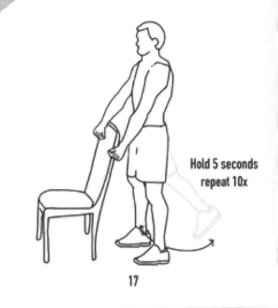

Hold 5 seconds repeat 10x

17

18 - TREE POSE

- Stand up and balance yourself on your right foot.
- Place the sole of your left foot against your ankle, shin, or thigh while lifting the heel of your left foot and angling it to the side.
- Put your hands in a posture that is convenient for you.
- Hold for as long as a minute.
- Do the other side similarly.

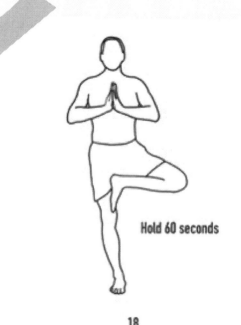

Hold 60 seconds

18

19 - MARCHING

- This marching drill can aid with balance and flexibility.
- Place your feet hip-width apart and stand tall.
- Lift your foot and until your thigh is parallel to the ground, gradually budge your knee.
- If you can't lift your thigh all the way up, don't stress about it; lift it as high as you can.
- You can hang onto the back of a chair if additional support is required.

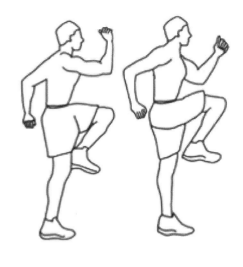

19

20 - STAIR TAPPING

- Place yourself in front of a step or a stool.
- For assistance, you can use a cane or side rail.
- Bring your left leg up to meet your right leg as you take a step forward.
- Then descend in the same order.
- Start over with the other leg and complete the cycle 15–20 times more.

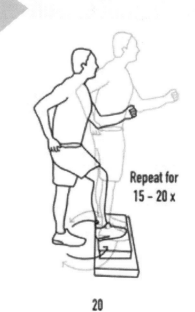

Repeat for
15 - 20 x

20

21 - ALTERNATING VISION WALKS

- Set your feet hip-width apart as you begin at one end of the space.
- Take four or five steps forward while keeping this head position and looking over your right shoulder.
- Observe your left shoulder for a moment and then move your head.
- Take a further four or five steps after that.
- Repeat five times on each side.

Affix a weight to your chest as you perform the workout for a more difficult variation.

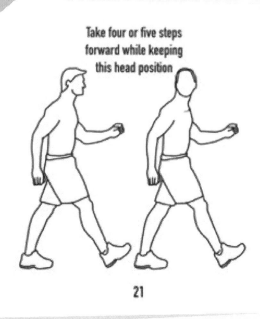

Take four or five steps forward while keeping this head position

21

22 - SIT-TO-STANDS

- Taking a position in front of a chair with your back facing the seat.
- Sit in the chair slowly.
- After taking a brief break, stand back up.
- Repeat ten times.

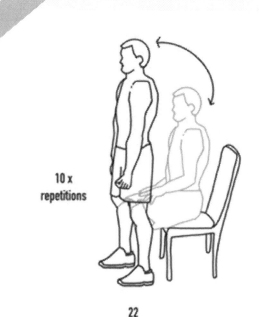

10 x repetitions

22

23 - FORWARD AND BACKWARD TILT

The balancing board is the best tool for this workout.

- Place your feet on the balance board's outer edges as you stand.
- Lean forward till the board's front touches the ground.
- Hold on to this position for a short while.
- Then, sag backward until the board's rear is in contact with the ground.
- Hold on to this position for a short while.

Continue back and forth slowly for one minute.

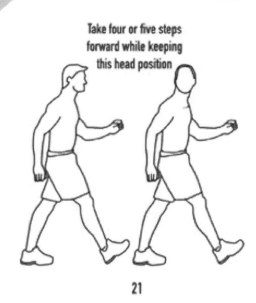

Take four or five steps forward while keeping this head position

21

24 - SEMI-TANDEM POSITION

- Standing with one foot's big toe inside the other's arch.
- Forward-facing toes.
- In close proximity for safety, a chair or rail.
- Hold for as long as you can—at least 30 seconds.
- Move on to the following position safely if you can hold for 30 seconds.

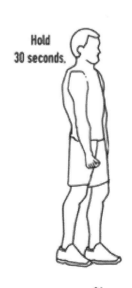

Hold 30 seconds.

24

25 - ALTERNATE FEET

- To begin, use a chair or countertop as a base of support.
- For 10 seconds, lift your right leg out to the side and maintain it there.
- Repeat for 10 to 15 circuits, switching legs each time.

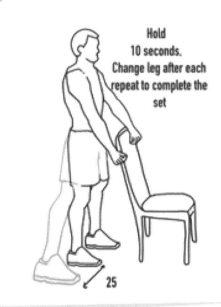

Hold 10 seconds. Change leg after each repeat to complete the set

25

26 - CHAIR LEG RAISES

- Straighten your back while you sit on a chair.
- Now raise your left leg to a height of 5 inches and maintain for 5 seconds.
- Repeat with your right leg, bringing your foot back to the ground.
- Keep up this "slow march" for three to five minutes.

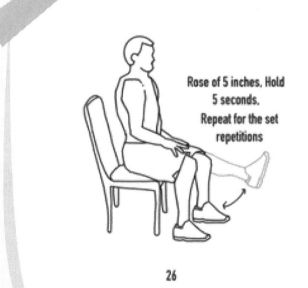

Rose of 5 inches. Hold 5 seconds. Repeat for the set repetitions

26

27 - UPPER BODY ROTATIONS

- Stand up and place your hands on your hips.
- Slowly forward-tilt your upper body from the hips.
- Make a full circle by rotating it to your right, backward, and left.
- Ten circles can be drawn with your upper torso.

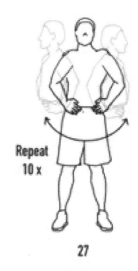

28 - BALL MARCHES

- Start by taking a comfortable seat on the ball.
- Stay focused in your center.
- In a leisurely march, start lifting each leg alternately a few inches above the ground.
- Do this for a minute or two.

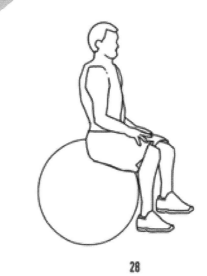

29 - SINGLE-LEG CROSS-BODY PUNCHES

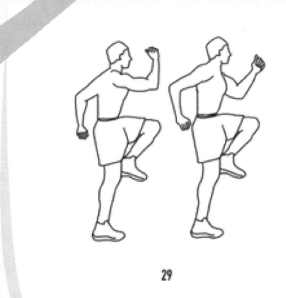

29

- To begin, stand on one leg.
- Punch slowly into the air, switching between the right and left arms.
- Move your upper body while engaging your core.

30 - THE COMPASS

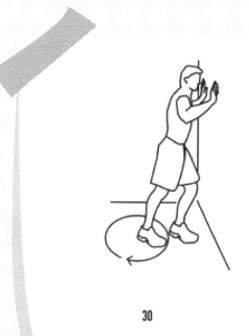

30

- To assist you, lean against a wall or something else.
- Your right leg must be behind you as your left knee is slightly bent.
- With your right leg, create arcs of circles, then carry out the motion repeatedly.
- This time, bend the right leg while you perform the exercise.

31 - BALANCING BEAM

- Align your right foot with your left and step forward until the heel hits the toes.
- Lift your left foot to the front, again touching the heel to the toes, and slowly move your weight to your right leg.
- Take this route for 20–30 steps.

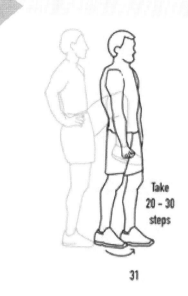

32 - LADDER

- If you don't have a rope ladder, you can draw one out or use your imagination if you don't have one to set it on the floor. This activity is frequently done during football practice.
- Your right leg should first enter each rung of the ladder, followed by your left.
- Then step out the same way.
- This should be done all the way up the ladder.

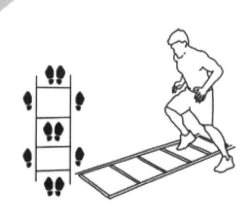

33 - SIT AND ROCK LATERALLY

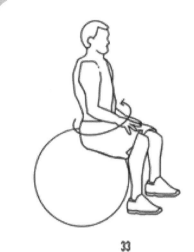

- Lay on an exercise ball with your forward-facing.
- As soon as you feel secure, start to rock your hip to the left and then back to the middle.
- For a total of three minutes, repeat this exercise to the right.

33

34 - BEACH BALL EQUILIBRIUM (WITH A PARTNER)

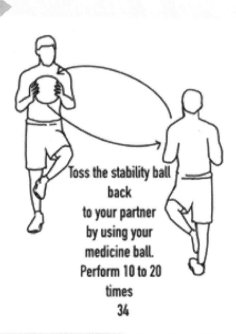

- Standing on one or both legs on a Bosu Balance Trainer's platform while holding a medicine ball.
- Ask your spouse to toss a stability ball in your direction.
- Toss the stability ball back to your partner by using your medicine ball.
- Perform 10 to 20 times.

Toss the stability ball back to your partner by using your medicine ball. Perform 10 to 20 times

34

35 - MOUNTAIN POSE

- Stand with your toes in contact and your heels a little apart.
- To activate the muscles in your lower legs, lift and spread your toes.
- Kneel slightly while maintaining core engagement.

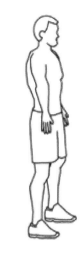

35

36 - SIDE PLANK POSE

- Lay on your left side with your feet together and your left forearm directly beneath your left shoulder to begin.
- Once your body is straight from head to toe, engage your core and lift your hips.
- Hold there for at least five breaths while continuing to breathe, keeping your hips from dropping.

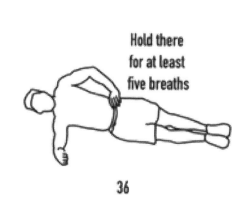

Hold there for at least five breaths

36

37 - FORWARD LUNGE WALK

- Standing is a good place to start. Steps: one foot forward and lunge.
- Knees over ankles, both legs bent at a 90-degree angle, and hold for a breath.
- To elevate and go back to standing, contract your inner thighs and activate your glutes.
- On the opposite side, repeat.
- For ten or more repetitions on each side, continue alternating.

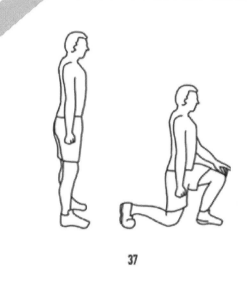

37

38 - PLANK WITH ELBOWS ON A STABILITY BALL

- Place your elbows and forearms on a stability ball and assume the plank position.
- Keep your hips and shoulders level while using your abdominal, glutes, and quadriceps to maintain appropriate alignment.
- Maintain this position for up to three seconds.

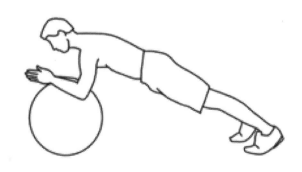

39 - BOSU DOG BIRD

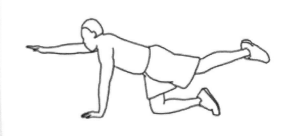

39

- Get on all fours and stand atop a flat-side-down Bosu. Your palms should be facing up, and your knees should be just below the middle. Your feet must be flat on the ground.
- Lift both the left arm and right leg simultaneously off the Bosu until they are parallel to the ground. Maintain a neutral neck and hip alignment with the ball.
- Lift the opposite arm and leg, then lower the first arm and leg back to the Bosu.
- Repeat ten times on each side.

40 - TOE BALANCE SQUAT

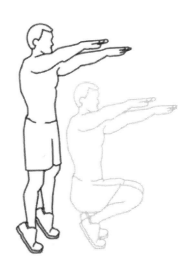

40

- Steps: forward with your toes touching and your heels a little apart.
- Knees should be slowly bent while thighs and heels are compressed.
- Lift your heels off the floor and squeeze your feet's balls down while maintaining an engaged core. Attempt to maintain a straight spine as you descend.

With your heels up, can you reach the ground all the way? Wherever you are, hold for ten breaths.

41 - SUMO SQUAT WITH OUTER THIGH PULSE

- Start with your feet 45 degrees out from the center.
- To lower into a sumo squat, bend at the hips and knees. Maintain a straight torso.
- Extend the other arm and one leg as you stand. Hold and extend your leg three times by two to three inches.
- Return your leg to the starting position, then do it again.
- Alternate sides for 12 reps.

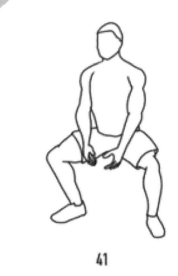

41

42 - CURTSY LUNGE WITH OBLIQUE CRUNCH

- Stand with your feet hip-width apart, your elbows out wide, and your fingertips near your ears.
- Lunging forward with one leg crossed behind you, curtsying.
- Standing, For an oblique crunch, raise that same leg up until it touches the same side elbow without rotating your hips.

After 12 repetitions, switch legs.

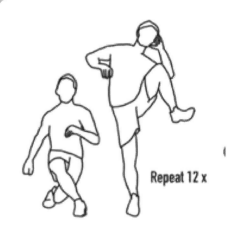

Repeat 12 x

42

43 - PLANK WITH FLYING PLANE ARMS

- Begin with your arms in a high plank position and your hands directly beneath your shoulders.
- Keep your hips firm and your core engaged as you raise one arm straight out in front of you.
- As you continue to hold it aloft, fan it out to the side.
- Bring your hand back to the front and then let it fall to the ground.
- Follow the same pattern on the opposite side.
- Alternate the sides continuously For 12 rounds.

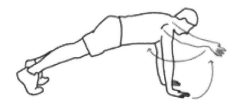

Repeat 12 x

43

44 - ROLLING FOREARM SIDE PLANK

- Start by supporting your body weight on one forearm in a side plank position. Put your shoes on top of one another. Lengthen the upper arm.
- Changing which arm is on the ground and which is in the air, roll to the opposite side of your body.
- Hold for two to three seconds on each side.
- Roll from side to side 12 more times.

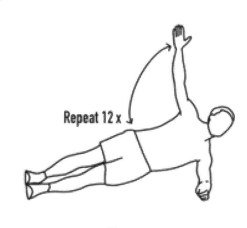

Repeat 12 x

44

45 - ARM SEQUENCE WITH LIFTED HEELS

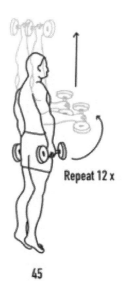

- Position your feet shoulder-width apart, your knees slightly bent, and your knees inwards pressed.
- Hold a set of light to medium dumbbells with your arms at your sides.
- Your heel lift needs to be increased by about two inches. Hold this posture as you execute a shoulder press and bicep curl.
- Maintaining an extended front arm position as you lower the weights to the starting position.
- Throughout the action, keep a tight core to prevent arching your back.
- Repeat Eight times through the series.

Repeat 12 x

45

46 - T-STAND WITH SIDE BEND AND HINGE

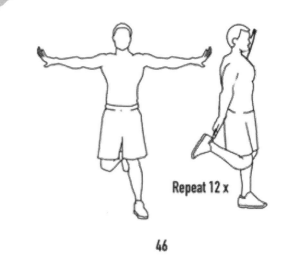

- With your hands out to the side and Keeping your right knee bent at a 90-degree angle, start standing on your left leg to balance.
- Lift your right leg up behind you as you hinge at the hips and engage your core.
- As you do so, bend your right elbow till it touches the inner of your left ankle.
- As you start, bring your right hand down until it lands outside your right leg.
- On one side, repeat the sequence eight times. Continue on the other side.

Repeat 12 x

46

47 - FLAMINGO STAND

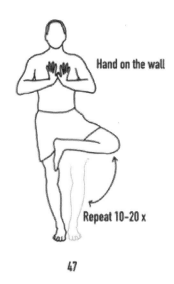

- Start by placing your hands on a wall while standing with your feet shoulder-width apart.
- Now lift your right leg up to your hip as though you were marching. Lower it, then lower the left, and repeat.
- You can make it more difficult by moving a little faster or lifting your legs higher.
- Repeat between 10 and 20 times for both sides.

Hand on the wall

Repeat 10-20 x

47

48 - BODY CIRCLE

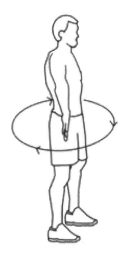

- Start by taking a tall stance and spreading your feet wide.
- Lean forward slightly while maintaining a stable lower body and a straight upper body.
- Slowly tilt your body in a circular motion to the left, back, and right.
- Avoid leaning too far to the back or the front.

48

49 - SEATED PILLOW SQUEEZES

- Place your arms at your sides and sit upright in a chair.
- Between your thighs or knees, place a pillow.
- By tensing the muscles in your inner thighs, squeeze the cushion.
- After three seconds, release the squeeze.
- Make 12 repetitions.

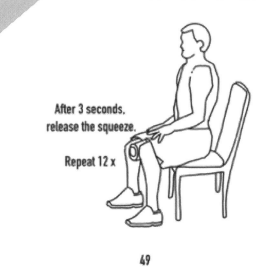

After 3 seconds,
release the squeeze.

Repeat 12 x

49

50 - SEATED CLAMSHELLS

- Place your arms at your sides and sit upright in a chair.
- Put your hands on the outside of your knees while bending your knees. The resistance for your legs will come from your hands.
- You can tighten the muscles around your hips by attempting to move your knees apart. Push your knees in a while doing this by applying resistance with your hands and arms.
- Three seconds into the contraction, release it.
- Make 12 repetitions.

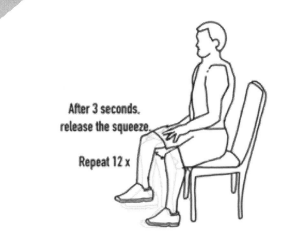

After 3 seconds,
release the squeeze.

Repeat 12 x

50

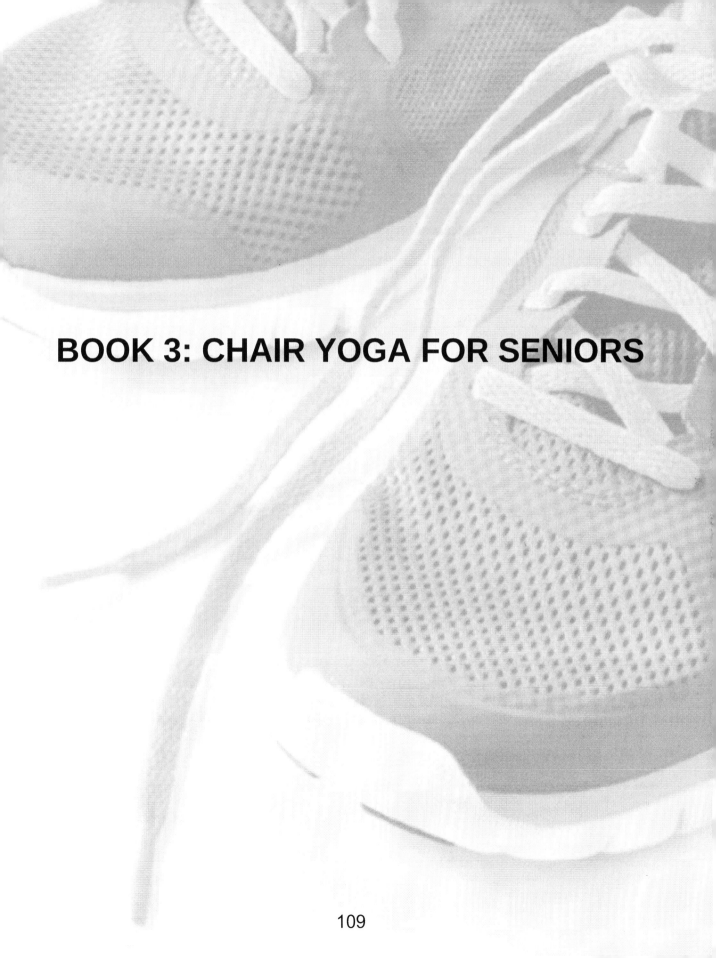

BOOK 3: CHAIR YOGA FOR SENIORS

To survive as we age, we must modify our routines and lives. Exercise can be more challenging if you have joint discomfort, sore muscles, weariness, or other age-related conditions. These worries frequently lead seniors to unproductive or sedentary lifestyles, worsening the situation. However, chair yoga is an easy and affordable type of exercise that has a lot of benefits for seniors.

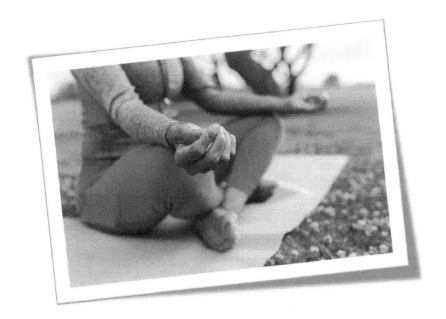

What is Yoga?

Yoga signifies the integration of the body and the mind. Yoga is a way of life that teaches us to be in the now and arouses our curiosity in the various levels of our being, including our physical, organic, physiological, psychological, pranic, emotional, and spiritual sensations. Additionally, the goal of yoga practice is to stop mental swings.

From a physical standpoint, yoga practice fosters flexibility and body awareness, boosts strength and balance, and may be beneficial for certain musculoskeletal issues. Yoga enhances joint mobility and corrects postural alignment. In addition to its physical advantages, Yoga has significant neurological effects. Yoga enables us to access the parasympathetic nerve system, which, among other things, aids in improved stress management, a calmer outlook on life, and more relaxed thinking. Additionally, Yoga teaches us several breathing practices that enable us to deepen and improve our breathing by becoming more conscious of it.

Yoga aids us in choosing the course of our thoughts, as the first four sutras of the Pantanji Yoga-Sutras suggest. Our genuine essence becomes apparent when the mind calms. Yoga teaches us how to control our thoughts to achieve inner quiet, stability, and tranquility.

The four paths of Yoga

1.Jnana Yoga – Yoga of knowledge, philosophy of Yoga

2.Bhakti Yoga – devotional Yoga, spiritual practices

3.Karma Yoga – yoga of selfless action, self-sacrifice

4.Raja Yoga – integral Yoga – The eight limbs of Yoga

Brief History of Yoga

Yoga is said to have been practiced since the dawn of humanity. The science of Yoga was created long before the first religions or belief systems were established. In yogic literature, Shiva is referred to as the first yogi, or Adiyogi, as well as the first Guru, or Adi Guru.

Most people think that Yoga is simply asanas and pranayamas used to maintain health. But this age-old discipline that aims to balance the body, mind, and spirit encompasses more than that. The English word "yoga" is derived from the Sanskrit word "yuj," which means "to link" or "to mix." It is intended to assist the person in overcoming hardship and advancing spiritually to the "state of liberation."

Yoga, one of the oldest sciences in existence, has its roots in India. In legend, Lord Shiva is credited with being the first to teach Yoga. An invention of the Indus valley civilization, Yoga dates back to 2700 BC and aims to advance humanity's physical and spiritual well-being. Yoga's core principles are fundamental human ideals. The Rig Veda has the oldest mention of "yoga." Since the Vedas were transmitted orally, it is impossible to pinpoint certain dates for the Atharva Veda's reference to "breath regulation."

But much earlier, about 2700 BC, the Indus-Saraswati culture produced many seals that showed yoga asanas. The Vedas, Upanishads, Smritis, teachings of Buddha, Panini, the epics, the Puranas, and other relevant literature are the primary sources that provide knowledge about Yoga and related literature.

The classical period, from 500 BC to 800 AD, is regarded as the most fruitful for the development of Yoga. During this time, Mahavira and Buddha both appeared as prominent religious figures, and Vyasa wrote his commentary on the Yoga Sutras. The classical period, from 500 BC to 800 AD, is regarded as the most fruitful for the development of Yoga. During this time, Mahavira and Buddha both appeared as prominent religious figures, and Vyasa wrote his commentary on the Yoga Sutras. You could think of Buddha's eight-fold path as the origin of yoga sadhana. The Bhagwad Gita discusses the concepts of Gyan Yoga, Bhakti Yoga, and Karma Yoga in greater detail and provides more in-depth explanations. They endure forever and still have value today.

In addition to focusing on several facets of Yoga, Patanjali's Yoga Sutras is known for describing the eight-fold path of Yoga.

During this time, Mahavira and Buddha both appeared as prominent religious figures, and Vyasa wrote his commentary on the Yoga Sutras. You could think of Buddha's eight-fold path as the origin of yoga sadhana. The Bhagwad Gita discusses the concepts of Gyan Yoga, Bhakti Yoga, and Karma Yoga in greater detail and provides more in-depth explanations. They endure forever and still have value today.

In addition to focusing on several facets of Yoga, Patanjali's Yoga Sutras is known for describing the eight-fold path of Yoga. During this time, the mind was the main emphasis; Yoga aims to unify the body and mind to achieve serenity.

The Post-Classical era spans the years 800 to 1700. Adi Shankaracharya and Ramanujacharya were the more notable contributors then, while the teachings of Suradasa, Mirabai, and Tulsidas also became more well-known. Matsyendranath, Gorkshanatha, Suri, Gheranda, and Shrinivasa Bhatt popularized Hatha yoga during this time.

Later, Swami Vivekananda introduced Yoga to the West in the middle of the nineteenth century. Ramana Maharshi, Ramakrishna Paramahansa, K Pattabhi Jois, and Paramahansa Yogananda all contributed to the development of Raja Yoga.

By demystifying Yoga and making it accessible to the common person, Shri Yogendraji made a significant contribution to the field. As a result, millions of people who had previously believed that mystics and recluses only practiced Yoga could now access Yoga.

This has been the long trip that Yoga has made into the twenty-first century. Yes, it has evolved and grown through the years, but its core —becoming self-aware—remains unchanged.

Yoga as A Way Of Life Today

As stated earlier, Yoga unites the body, mind, and soul; it is more than just a collection of asanas. It is a highly scientific discipline with a deep understanding of maintaining one's physical fitness and tranquil, collected thought processes. It explains what to eat, how to eat, when to consume, and what to stay away from. Yogic science and Ayurveda are complementary disciplines. Ayurveda promotes healthy food and a way of life; it is a religious aspect of our Indian history, and incorporating Yoga into our daily routine is urgently needed.

The entire world is going through a difficult time, and we are all suffering the same or related difficulties. The ideal time to return to our roots is right now. The globe is embracing Yoga and transitioning to a much more holistic way of living, so we should investigate it. One of the key advantages of yoga and wellness practices is that they have no negative side effects and promote mental and physical health, all of which are crucial during this pandemic. They also have no adverse impacts on our bodies or minds.

Meditation, a component of Yoga that promotes emotional and mental health, is another practice. When everyone around you is experiencing tension and anxiety, meditation can help you take control of your thoughts. Your breathing serves as the link that joins your body and mind. You can easily control the mind if you master the ability to control your breath. You can achieve a profoundly calm state while meditation, a deep slumber that is frequently more effective than sleeping. It's been suggested that 20 minutes of meditation is equivalent to four hours of sleep in terms of its health effects.

Through meditation, you can access your inner world and come to understand that your happiness and joy come from within. Numerous studies have demonstrated the benefits of Yoga and meditation. Yoga has started to be taught in most universities all over the world. The world is embracing a holistic way of life and practicing mindfulness. These insights come from India. This information must be preserved; it is both our own and our duty to share it with everyone around the globe. This was a truly exceptional choice as it significantly contributed to raising public awareness of this treatment.

What is chair yoga for seniors?

All people can perform seniors chair yoga, which only calls for a basic chair. It enables gentle yoga practice! The elderly and working persons who want to practice at their place of employment are its target audiences. It is a fantastic option if you have pain that prevents you from engaging in traditional Yoga.

As a result, a chair can be used to support a variety of traditional postures. The chair merely supports the body. It simply takes the place of the mat and turns into a true yoga item. This seated yoga exercise improves posture, tones muscles, and lowers stress levels. It also lessens persistent discomfort, including back pain, and helps to soften particular body parts. Physical activity is crucial for maintaining a high quality of life as one age. When we reach the age of 60, we need to switch up the kind of discipline we practice because high-impact sports like running, cycling, and swimming lose their functional benefits. Seniors who practice chair Yoga may find this to be the solution.

Five Equipment's for Chair Yoga

Although chair yoga is a low-risk and low-impact exercise, you need the proper equipment to save and maximize your performance. Among the necessary chair yoga equipment are:

1.An armless, stable chair

2.A flat, level surface for your chair

3.Clothing that is flexible and comfortable but not overly tight or baggy

4.Enough room to spread your limbs fully

5.An experienced instructor or friend for safety

7 Benefits Of Chair Yoga For Seniors

It's no secret that exercise provides a variety of advantages that endure long into your senior years, but doing high-intensity workouts as the body ages and gets more fragile poses a risk. The likelihood of suffering pain and injury is high, and recovery takes longer. You may start exercising more generally with Yoga without running the danger of strains.

Let's examine the advantages of chair yoga, which uses a chair for support since numerous older people generally do Yoga. For instance, those with movement difficulties, arthritis, vertigo, and other conditions can benefit greatly from chair yoga.

1.Increased Flexibility

Yoga is known for its ability to increase flexibility, and chair yoga is no exception. Chair yoga encourages the body to push itself while stretching areas that might not typically be stretched. This improves people's general mobility for daily chores by helping them retain and grow their flexibility.

2.   Improves Muscle Strength

Muscles can be strengthened and built through various chair yoga poses. This aids in enhancing balance and movement, coupled with flexibility. Gaining strength will also assist in keeping your body injury-free.

3.   Helps with Balance and Coordination

Through changing poses, chair yoga helps your body become more spatially aware.

Yoga teaches you to pay attention to and use all the different areas of your body, making you feel closer to your physical self. You gradually get better coordination and balance training from doing this.

4. Improves pain management techniques and reduces pain

Every time you exercise, a hormone called endorphins is created, which not only contributes to an improvement in your positive mood but also helps to lessen some of the pain and suffering. By concentrating on your breathing, chair yoga teaches you how to manage pain while drawing on the body's natural medications.

5. Improves Sleep Quality

Regular exercise improves the quality of your sleep while regulating your body's sleep-wake cycle. The same is true of chair yoga since it requires just the correct amount of energy without making you feel exhausted.

6. Increases Self-Assurance and Reduces Depression and Anxiety

According to research, people of all ages can benefit from Yoga, including chair yoga, in reducing their feelings of anxiety and despair. You can eliminate any unfavorable feelings from life by using the focus required for Yoga, and you'll feel lighter and more refreshed afterward.

7. Better proprioception, coordination, and balance:

The awareness of your body's movements in space is known as proprioception; as you move from one pose to the next in a chair yoga sequence, your proprioception increases, which will improve your balance and coordination all around.

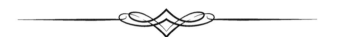

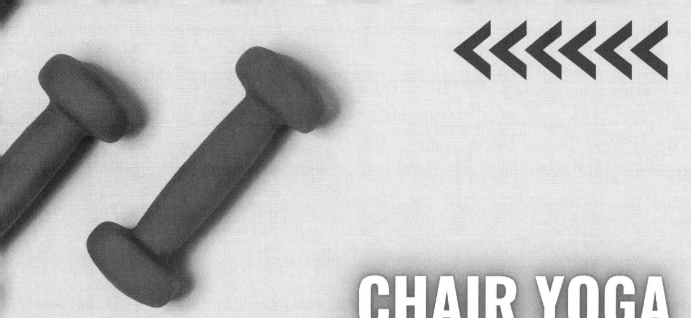

CHAIR YOGA
FOR SENIORS

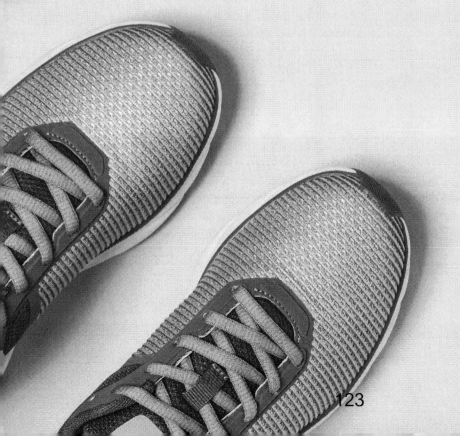

PART 3

Easy Exercises

1 - EAGLE POSE

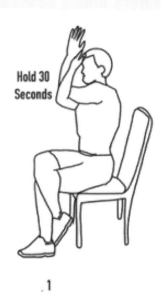

Hold 30 Seconds

- Seat and maintain a straight, toned back.
- Overlap the left and right legs. Bring the right foot forward, and wrap the left foot around the right shin if you can.
- Hold the arms forward at a 90-degree angle and cross the left elbow over the right elbow, pointing upwards with their fingers.
- Stretching your head upward while keeping your shoulders far from your ears.
- Repeat three times while maintaining this stance for around 30 seconds.

.1

2 - THE CATTLE-CAT

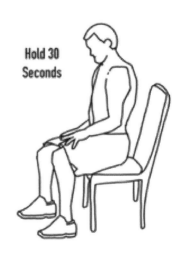

Hold 30 Seconds

- Put your hands on your knees as you sit down.
- Inhale deeply while gazing up at the sky.
- Raise your shoulders away from your ears, push your chest forward, and pinch your shoulder blades together.
- Then let out a breath and raise your arms.
- Bring the chin to the neck while maintaining the round back.

2

3 - DOWNWARD DOG POSE

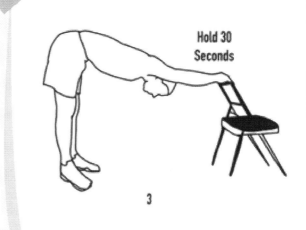

Hold 30 Seconds

- Face your chair while standing. Leg distance should be at least shoulder width.
- Put your hands on the chair's top and firmly press down.
- As soon as your back is straight, take a few steps back. Your buttocks should be as stretched up towards the ceiling as you can. Your shoulders align with the width of your hands, which are firmly planted on the chair. The spine continues into the head.
- Breathe slowly, and if necessary, stoop to your knees. This will shield the lower back from harm and discomfort.
- Finish by approaching the chair and slowly rising.

4 - PALM TREE POSE OR THE ARMS-UP POSE

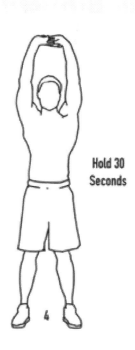

Hold 30 Seconds

- Keep your body in a natural position with a straight back, relaxed shoulders, and a forward-facing chest.
- Place the chair's arms on the sides. These ought to stretch out completely and fall naturally.
- The feet must be positioned with their customary openness, parallel to the front.
- Make a gradual rise in front of you by raising your arms without bending your elbows. After a brief period, leave them at the top before returning to your starting position.
- You can alternate this arm raise with raises from the flanks if you'd like.

5 - DOVE POSE

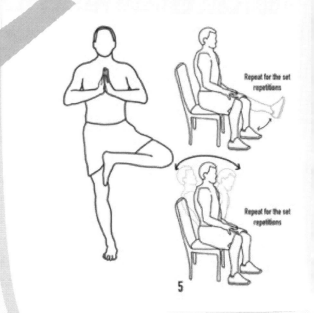

- Raise your left leg such that the ankle rests on your right leg while you sit naturally.
- Try to lift the leg with the knee aligned with the ankle as much as possible; this will create a straight line parallel to the ground.
- Hold this leg with the natural shoulder opening while keeping your arms straight.
- Swing your torso back and forth, keeping your back in mind. It must stay tension-free and straight.

6 - HALF TWIST POSE

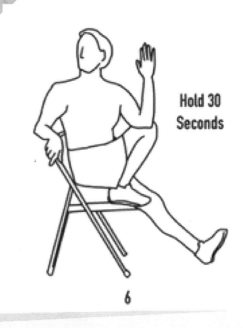

Hold 30 Seconds

- Your entire body should be pointing to the right as you sit sideways on the chair.
- Bring your feet together, extend your back in a straight stance, and tense your abdominal muscles.
- Turn your upper body slowly so your face faces the chair's back.
- Keep your feet on the ground as much as possible, and maintain a static hip position.
- To finish the motion, you can hold the backrest. After maintaining this strain for a few seconds, return to your starting posture.
- Apply these similar techniques to the other side of your body after performing 5–10 reps on one side.

7 - WARRIOR POSTURE

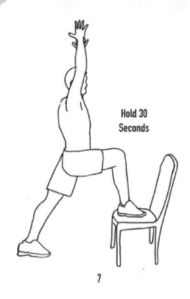

Hold 30 Seconds

- Place your right leg sideways so that the biceps femoris, the lower portion of the thigh, rests on the seat. The foot should be entirely in contact with the ground, and the calf should form a vertical line.
- The other leg, the left, must be extended backward until it forms a straight line. In this situation, you should only have your toes on the ground.
- Reach your arms up and bring your hands together while keeping your torso solid and your back straight.
- Once you've held it for a few seconds, switch sides

8 - TENSE SIDE ANGLE

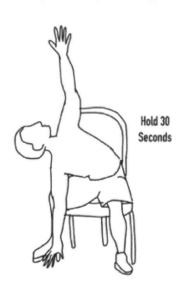

Hold 30 Seconds

- With your arms by your sides and in a natural stance, sit.
- Turn your body to the left, stooping forward, and place your right hand's palm on the ground. The base of contact should be a few inches above your left foot, with the arm fully extended.
- Your attention should be focused on the left arm, which should be the other arm, and fully stretched upward.
- When performing this move, your back needs to be protected. Make sure it's straight and doesn't create any unnecessary tension.

Switch sides to engage the muscles on the opposite side after maintaining this position for a few seconds.

9 - PLIERS

- With your arms outstretched, sit in the starting posture.
- Lean forward gently with the body. Pay attention to your back during this procedure and keep your focus fixed on it as you drop.
- Keep your body in this position for a few seconds while making sure your palms are in contact with the ground.
- Your arms should be fully extended, your shoulders should be forward, and your heels should not be off the ground.

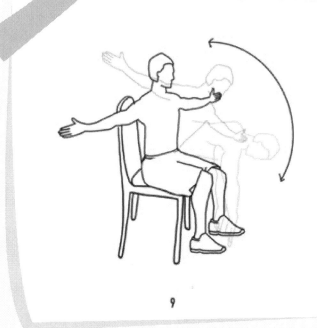

9

10 - SEATED SUPINE TWIST

- Sit in the mountain with us.
- Pointing your fingers forward, extend both hands out in front of you.
- Exhale while inhaling and, as you do so, twist at the waist, turning your hands and completing the torso to the right.
- 2–3 breaths should be held.
- Go to the left and then back to the middle.

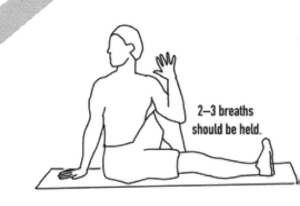

2–3 breaths should be held.

10

11 - TRIANGLE POSITION

- Stand in front of the chair.
- Your left leg takes a backward step of about 3-2 feet with the right foot.
- The right foot should remain forward.
- With fingers pointing out to the sides, spread both hands.
- Lean forward till your right hand is resting on the edge of the chair while loading your right hip joint.
- Press the right hip forward and open the left hip, turning it outward and back to align your hips.
- Lift the left hand and aim it upwards.
- Press your feet together while maintaining both knees straight, using a micro-elbow if necessary.
- You can either raise your hand, look up, or straight ahead.

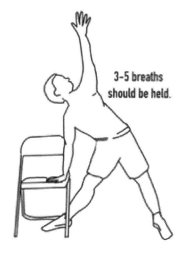

3-5 breaths should be held.

11

12 - DANCER POSE

- Pose behind the chair's back while seated on the mountain.
- Both hands should be on the backrest.
- Pressing into the corners of the feet and raising the kneecap to activate the quadriceps will secure the right leg.
- Reach the inner of the left foot with your left hand by raising the left leg back.
- As you lift, kick your left foot back.
- As you stretch the sides of the body, lengthen the torso by pulling in your abdomen and rib cage.
- Keep your leg straight, or bend it just slightly behind the knees.
- As you lift your chest, pull your shoulder blades back and downward.

Lengthen the neck, maintain a firm posture, and look ahead. Hold for 3-5 breaths and switch sides.

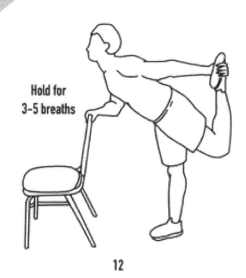

Hold for 3-5 breaths

12

13 - GODDESS POSE WITH A TWIST

- Sit on your chair in tadasana.
- To straddle the seat, spread your legs widely.
- The right foot and knee should face the right side, while the left foot and knee should face the left side.
- Lengthen your torso and ground your sit bones.
- With your fingers pointed up toward the ceiling, extend both of your hands.
- Bend to the left while maintaining an elongated body. Place the left hand on the floor with the fingertips pointing down and the elbow resting against the left leg. You can use a bock to support your left hand.
- Look at the raised right hand.
- ØHold for 3-5 breaths.
- Switch sides.

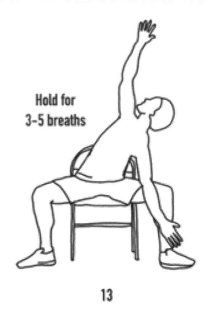

Hold for
3~5 breaths

13

14 - PIGEON POSE

- Sitting in tadasana.
- Knees and feet should be hip-width separated.
- Place the left angle above the right knee while lifting the left leg and bending the knees.
- Lengthen your torso and tilt forward at the hip.
- Hold for 3 to 5 breaths while looking forward.
- Change sides.
- High alter side lean,
- lift your arm, and interlace your fingers in front of you.
- Turn your palm into the ceiling as you straighten your arm above your head.

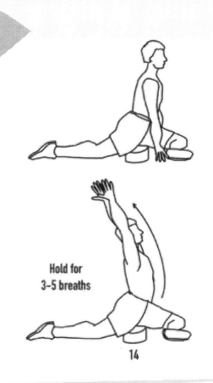

Hold for
3-5 breaths

14

15 - FORWARD BEND

- Sit on a chair in tadasana.
- Lean forward while keeping your tummy and chest on the thighs by hingeing at the hip joint.
- On your knees, let your head hang.
- Put your hands on the ground, palms or fingertips down.
- Hold for 3-5 breaths.

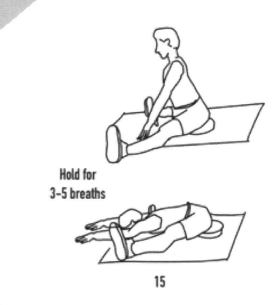

Hold for
3-5 breaths

15

16 - TWISTED-SPINE POSE

- Maintain proper posture while leaning back on the edge of your chair.
- Lengthen your spine as you inhale.
- Exhale while turning your torso to the left and reaching for the chair's back with your left arm.
- Repeat on the opposite side

Breathe ten times on each side, then switch.

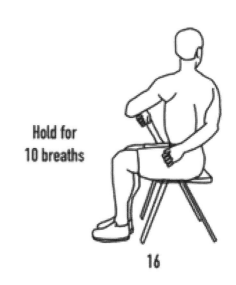

Hold for
10 breaths

16

17 - EXTENDED SIDE ANGLE POSE

- Start in the Seated Forward Fold but move your left hand's fingertips to the outside of your left foot instead. If you can't reach the floor, use a block.
- As you take a breath, turn your torso to the right. Open your chest as you raise your right arm and look up toward the ceiling.
- Hold for a number of deep breaths.
- On an out-breath, lower your back into the Forward Fold when you're ready.
- Repeat on the opposite side.

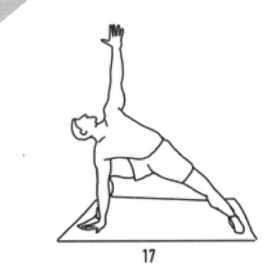

17

18 - FIREFLY POSE

- From Mountain Pose, extend your knees wide toward the chair's seat corners.
- Put your hands on the seat's front edge so they are comfortable.
- As though you were going to raise your body off the chair like in Firefly, lengthen your spine, contract your abs, and firmly press your hands into the chair seat.

Straighten both of your legs by contracting your thighs, then lift your feet off the ground

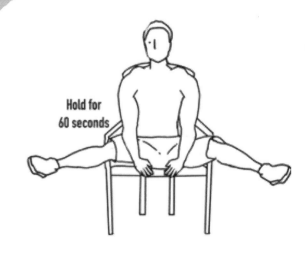

Hold for 60 seconds

18

19- STANDING HALF FORWARD BEND

- Standing two to three feet in front of a chair, face it.
- When you exhale, bend forward at the hips until your back is parallel to the ground. Put your hands on the chair's seat.
- Lift your navel toward your spine, raise your shoulders away from your ears, and extend your head forward to lengthen your spine.
- Look directly down.
- Return to standing when you're ready to do so.

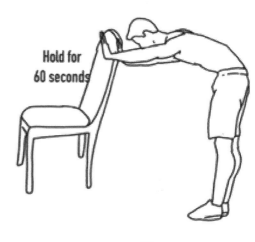

Hold for 60 seconds

19

20 - SPHINX

- With your elbows tucked under your shoulders, lie on your stomach and rest your forearms on the mat.
- Draw your shoulder blades together, down your back, and firmly into your arms.

Inhale deeply and hold the position for five to eight breaths.

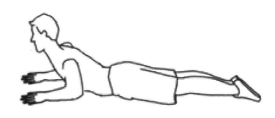

21 - THE COBBLER'S POSE

- As you open your knees to the sides, sit tall and bring the soles of your feet together.
- Fold forward to get a deeper stretch, but watch out for rounding your lower back too much.
- Take five to eight breaths while holding.

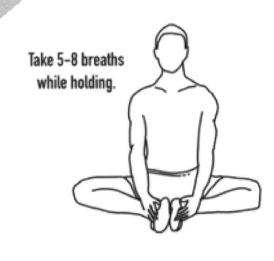

Take 5-8 breaths while holding.

21

22 - SAVASANA

- Lay on the ground and let it support you.
- As you lay there, take a long, restorative breath and completely relax your muscles.

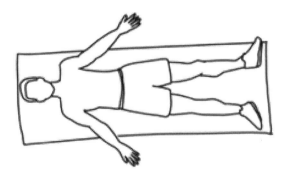

22

23 - DOG BIRD

- Begin by bending at the knees and extending one arm and the opposite leg forward. Draw your belly button toward your spine like a teacup resting on your back.
- Continue for a moment, then switch sides.
- Repeat five times.

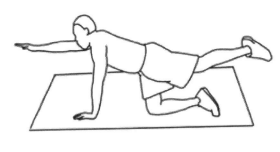

23

24 - STANDING PINCER POSTURE

- While standing, join the palms of the hands to stretch the arms later forward and slowly tilt the torso until it touches the floor or the knees.

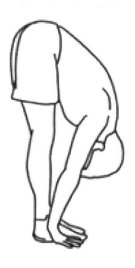

24

25 - CHAIR SUN WORSHIPPER

- Place yourself in the chair's front row and both feet flat on the floor
- Draw your arms back and curl your fingers over the back edge of the chair seat
- Inhale, squeeze your shoulder blades together, and lift up through your chest
- Exhale, drop your head back (if it's okay with your neck)
- Stay in this position for 3-4 breaths
- Come back to the center and then repeat one more time.

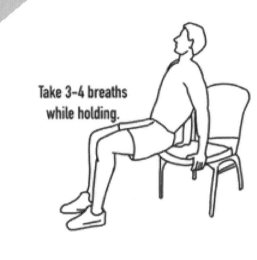

Take 3-4 breaths while holding.

25

26 - CHAIR STRADDLE FORWARD FOLD

- Start sitting up tall
- Spread feet apart so they are a little wider than the base of the chair, with your toes pointing forward.
- ØFold forward, and hold onto your ankles.
- Inhale, lift your chest slightly, and lengthen through the spine
- Exhale and fold forward, pulling against your ankles to fold a little deeper
- Let your head and neck relax completely
- Stay in this position for 3-4 breaths
- Slowly come back up to sitting.

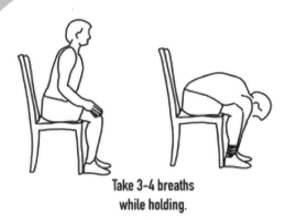

Take 3-4 breaths while holding.

26

27 - CHAIR HAMSTRING STRETCH (ONE LEG AND DOUBLE LEG)

- Sit tall, facing forward, with both feet flat on the floor.
- Extend your right leg, straightening your knee and placing your heel on the floor with your toes flexed up towards the ceiling.
- Inhale, sit up tall with your hands placed on your thighs.
- Exhale, reach your chest forward, and press back through your sitting bones as you hinge forward at your hips.
- Relax your head and neck.
- Stay in this position for 3-4 breaths.
- Slowly come back up to sitting.
- Repeat on the other side.

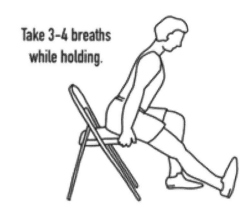

Take 3-4 breaths while holding.

27

28 - CHAIR LEG LIFT

- ØSit tall, facing forward, with both feet flat on the floor.
- ØExtend your right leg, straightening your knee and placing your heel on the floor with your toes flexed up towards the ceiling.
- ØInhale, sit up tall with your hands placed on your thighs.
- ØExhale, and lift your right leg off the floor.
- ØStay in this position for 3-4 breaths.
- Repeat on the other side.

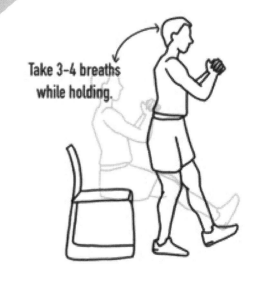

Take 3-4 breaths while holding.

28

29 - CHAIR COW'S FACE

- Sit tall and place your feet firmly on the ground.
- Inhale, and reach your right arm up.
- Bend your right elbow and drop your right hand down your back
- Bring your left arm out to the side with your palm turned back
- Bend your left elbow and reach your left hand up your back until it connects with your right hand
- If your hands don't reach each other, use a strap to bridge the gap and help you to work your hands toward each other.
- Stay in this position for 3-4 breaths
- Repeat on the other side

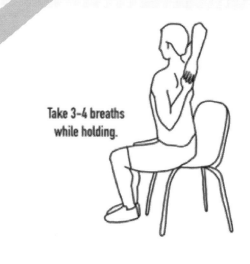

Take 3-4 breaths while holding.

29

30 - CHAIR SUN SALUTATION

- Place your feet flat on the floor while seated.
- Inhale, reach arms overhead, and slightly arch back
- Exhale, fold forward, bringing hands towards feet or hold opposite elbows
- Inhale, bring hands to ankles or shins, and lift head and chest to lengthen through the spine
- Exhale, fold forward
- Inhale, sweep your arms overhead as you come back up to sitting
- Exhale, bring hands to heart
- Repeat this process 3 or 4 times

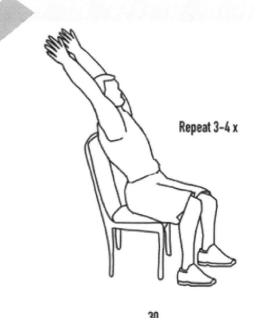

Repeat 3-4 x

30

138

31 - CHAIR FORWARD FOLD TWIST

- Bring your left hand to the floor next to your left foot as you fold forward while seated.
- Open your chest as you twist to the right on an inhale, bringing your right hand and gaze up towards the ceiling.
- Stay here for 3-4 breaths.
- Bring the right hand down on an exhale.
- Repeat on the other side. Repeat on both sides one more time.
- If your hand won't reach the floor, bring it to your forearm to your thigh instead (or use a block on the floor) and twist from there.
- For a more intense stretch, bring your hand to the opposite foot on the floor before twisting.

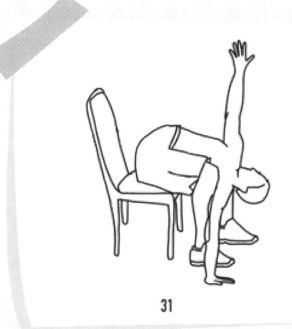

31

32 - CHAIR WARRIOR 2

- Start in Chair Warrior 1 (right foot in front)
- Exhale, turn the torso to the left, and open the arms with the right arm in front and the left arm going back.
- Keep looking forward over the right hand.
- Check that shoulders are directly over hips (not forward or back)
- Stay in this position for 3-4 breaths
- Go into the rest of the Warrior series from here, then repeat on the other side.

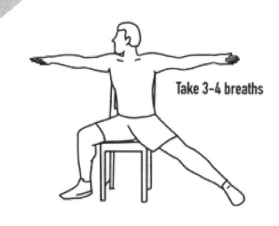

Take 3-4 breaths

32

33 - CHAIR REVERSE WARRIOR

- From Warrior 2 (right knee bent, right foot forward), drop the left arm down the back of the left leg.
- Lift the right arm up to the ceiling
- Stay in this position for 3-4 breaths
- Go into the rest of the Warrior series from here, then repeat on the other side.

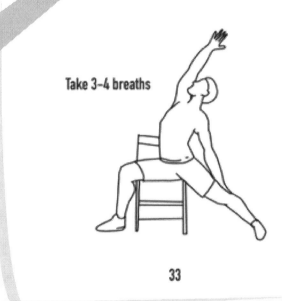

Take 3-4 breaths

33

34 - WARRIOR 3 WITH CHAIR

- Start standing, facing the chair.
- Steps: back about two feet away from the chair
- Place your hands around the sides of the chair
- Begin to straighten your arms and legs as you lift your right leg up
- Stay in this position for 3-4 breaths
- Exhale, lower your leg back to the floor
- Repeat on the other side.

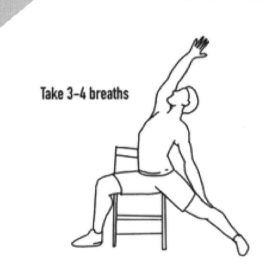

Take 3-4 breaths

33

140

35 - HALF MOON WITH CHAIR

- Start standing with your right side facing the chair
- Put your right hand in the center of the chair while bending your right knee.
- Breath, lift your left leg off the floor and lift your left-hand overhead
- Stay in this position for 3-4 breaths.
- Exhale, lower your arm, and lower your left foot back to the floor
- Turn to the other side and repeat on your other side

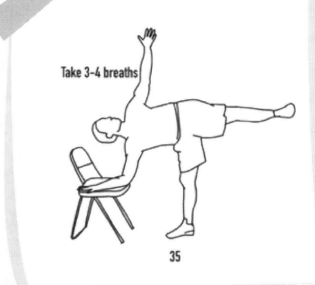

Take 3-4 breaths

35

36 - CHAIR LOCUST

- Place both of your feet down on the ground and sit forward in the chair.
- Fold forward, bringing your belly onto your thighs.
- Inhale, lift your head and chest, and Pull your shoulder blades together as you draw your arms back.
- Press your shoulders back away from your ears and breathe slowly
- Stay in this position for 3-4 breaths
- Slowly lower back to forward fold
- Repeat this posture one or two more times

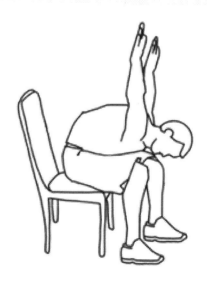

36

141

37 - CHAIR SPINAL TWIST

- Sit tall, facing forward, with both feet flat on the floor.
- Place the outside of your right knee with your left hand.
- Put your right hand on the chair's back.
- Inhale, sit up tall.
- Exhale, look over your right shoulder, and twist to the right.
- Stay in this position for 3-4 breaths.
- Continue to twist to the right, and then look over your left shoulder with your head turned.
- Stay in this position for 3-4 breaths.
- Release your hands and turn back to face forward.

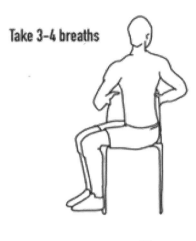

Take 3-4 breaths

37

38 - FINAL RELAXATION

- If you want to stay seated for final relaxation, place a bolster or folded blanket across your thighs.
- Rest your hands on the blanket or bolster with your palms up
- Gently close your eyes
- Sit tall, stacking your head and torso directly over your hips
- Breath in through your nose and exhale through your mouth
- Let the muscles in your face and shoulders relax completely
- Let your breathing become relaxed and natural, and follow the rhythm of your breath with your mind.
- Stay in this relaxed state for a couple of minutes
- Slowly open your eyes and stretch your arms overhead.

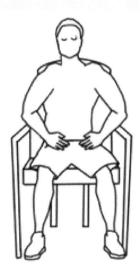

38

39 - EASY TWIST WHILE RECLINING

- Lie on your back with your legs spread and your knees bent.
- Lift your hips and move them to the left as you firmly plant your feet into the ground.
- Place your right hip underweight.
- Extend your arms with your palms facing up from your shoulders to around shoulder height.
- Rolling onto your right hip, bring your knees in toward your chest and drop them to the right. Your left shoulder blade should be extended toward the ground.
- Place your right hand on your left thigh to help your knees sink toward the floor.
- You can finish the twist by glancing at your left hand, the ceiling, or to the right.
- Hold the position for three to five minutes while taking deep breaths.
- Lift your knees to the center and take your hand off your thigh to release. Put pressure on your feet, then bring your hips back to the middle.
- Observe the effect of the stance while pausing to breathe.
- Repeat on the other side.

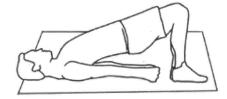
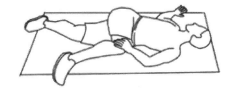

40

40 - CRESCENT STRETCH

- Place both of your feet firmly on the ground while sitting up straight.
- Place your left hand around the front of your right thigh.
- Inhale, and reach your right arm up next to your ear. Exhale and stretch to the left side while keeping your right arm next to your right ear.
- Open your chest towards the ceiling.
- Stay in this position for 3-4 deep breaths.
- Come back up and drop both hands next to your sides.
- Repeat on the other side.

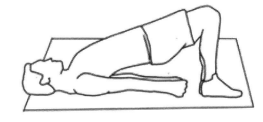
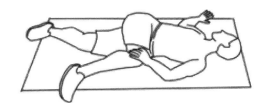

41 - MODIFIED BRIDGE POSE

- Set up shop on the floor in a sitting position.
- With your feet flat on the ground, squat down and bend your knees so they point upward. Directly over your knees should be a stack of your knees.
- Place a block, bolster, or folded blanket under your sacrum to raise your pelvis off the floor.
- Place your hands next to your body with the palms up, and release the weight of your pelvis onto the support.
- Pull your shoulder blades down and your shoulders away from your ears to place the weight of your shoulders on the floor.
- For additional support, you might tuck a tiny blanket under your neck.
- Let your neck stretch by lifting your chin away from the collars.
- Contemplate.
- Maintain the posture for five to ten breaths.

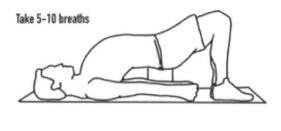

Take 5-10 breaths

41

42 - 3-WAY STANDING KICKS

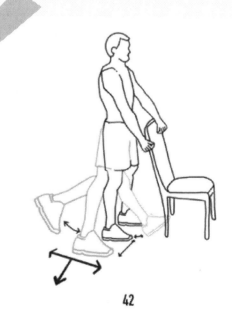

- Slowly extend the second leg in front of you while standing on one leg.
- Return your extended leg to the middle while keeping it as straight as you can.
- The same leg should be softly raised to the side, brought back down, and finally extended behind your body.
- Perform this in each direction.

42

43 - UJJAYI BREATHING

- Place your hands on your waist and lean back in your chair.
- Inhale deeply through your nose, allowing your sides and belly to stretch.
- Inhale deeply through your nose, allowing your sides and belly to stretch.
- Repeat ten times.

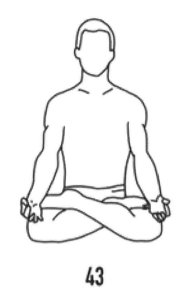

43

44 - PRAYER POSE

- Exhale and release your hands, and bring the palms together on the chest.
- Stand straight with your feet together.
- This is one full round of Sun Salutation.

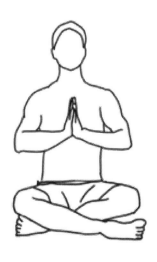

44

45 - REVOLVED SIDE ANGLE STRETCH

- Stand erect with the feet widely spread apart,
- Inhale, and turn the left foot to the left side.
- Exhale, bend your left knee, bend forward, rotate your trunk, bring your palms together and place your right elbow on the outer side of your left knee.
- Expand your chest up.
- Hold this pose for five breaths.
- Inhale, and release the hands to the front.
- Exhale and return to the starting position.
- Repeat on the other side.

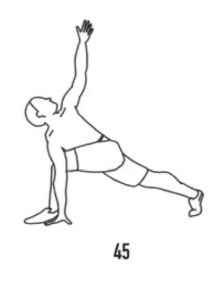

45

46 - CHEST EXPAND

- Stand erect with the feet widely spread apart.
- Inhale, raise both your hands up and tilt to the back.
- Expand the chest and hold it for a few seconds.
- Exhale, release the hands and return to the starting position.

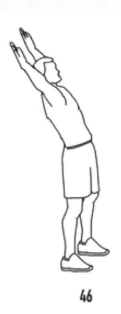

46

47 - EASY WARRIOR POSE III

- Exhale, lower your left knee, and bend the trunk forward.
- Rest the chest on the thigh and bring your hands forward.
- Keep the arms straight and the palms together.
- Hold this position for five long breaths.
- Exhale, lower your hands to the knee and raise up while straightening both your legs.
- Go back to starting position.
- Repeat on the right side.

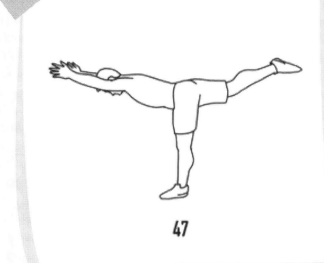

47

48 - HALF LOTUS POSE

- Sit with legs straight in front of the body.
- Bend one leg and place the sole of the foot on the inside of the opposite thigh.
- Bend the other leg and place the foot on top of the opposite thigh.
- Try to place the upper heel as near as possible to the abdomen without any strain.
- Adjust the position so that it is comfortable.
- Place your hands on your knees and close your eyes.
- Keep the head, neck and back upright and straight.
- Relax the whole body.
- Arms should be relaxed and not held straight.

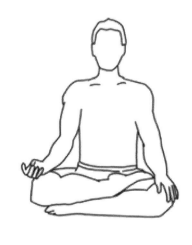

48

49 - LOTUS POSE

- Sit with legs straight in front of the body.
- Bend the left knee and place the left foot on the right thigh.
- Bend the right knee and place the right foot on the left thigh.
- Adjust the pose so that it is comfortable; the knees should be firmly on the floor.
- Place your hands on your knees and close your eyes.
- Keep the head, neck and back upright and straight.
- Relax the whole body.
- Arms should be relaxed and not held straight.

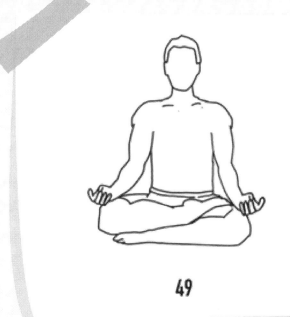

49

50 - THUNDERBOLT POSE I

- Kneel on the floor with the knees close together.
- Bring the big toes together and separate the heels.
- Lower the buttocks onto the inside surface of the feet with the heels.
- Touching the sides of the hips.
- Place the hands on the thighs, palms down.
- The back and head should be straight but not tense.
- Close the eyes, relax the arms and the whole body.

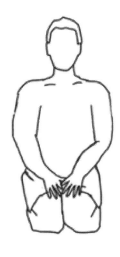

50

CONCLUSION

Whatever activity one is engaged in, be it Yoga or any other form, should provide contentment, satisfaction, and self-confidence. Learn to maintain a youthful mind, cultivate flexibility, strengthen the immune system, nourish the body, and much more. As one begins to reverse the biological age, tapping into the inner reservoirs of unlimited energy, creativity, and vitality becomes easy and natural, improving well-being. Yoga certainly helps change the habits of thinking and behaving and alters the experience of the body and the aging process. Teaching seniors is quite a challenge and a pleasure. Motivating them to regular practice takes a lot of work initially. But once they start over, there is nothing that can stop them. Their enthusiasm is quite a contagion. They need to feel important and that people give their undivided attention to them. Once the confidence is gained, they are easy and relaxed.

Their determination, commitment, and life experiences teach a very silent, salient, valuable lesson. This requires a lot of patience from the teacher's side.

But it is worth seeing their faces beaming with big confident smiles!!! Old age can be made not only bearable but also pleasurable. After all, old age is not a matter of years but a condition of mind, and Yoga brings a healthy state of mind. Yoga aims at enabling the individual to attain and maintain the "Sukhasthanam," which allows one to achieve physical, mental, and spiritual well-being. Yoga may not only add a few years to life but also may add life to the years. Therefore, the practice of Yoga should become an integral part of old age.

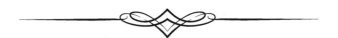

AFTERWORDS

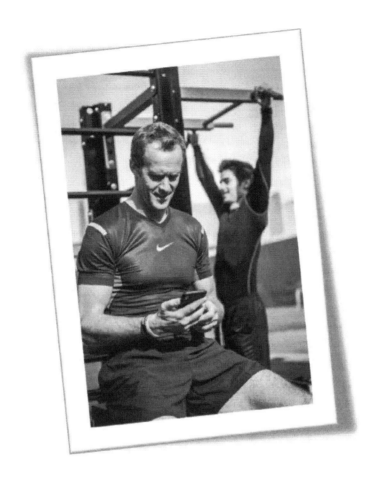

An individual's physical health, cognitive function, and psychological well-being may improve with frequent physical activity. Improvements in physical functioning, fitness, and overall quality of life are just a few of the physical advantages, but there are many more. There is evidence in the literature that exercise has cognitive benefits for aging, brain function, and academic performance.

Physical activity has psychological advantages, such as elevating mood and self-esteem and perhaps lowering stress, anxiety, and sadness. According to substantial scientific data, adopting a physical activity routine may have a good impact on health. However, people respond to exercise differently and may experience particular difficulties and barriers while starting and sticking with an exercise program. To increase physical activity, one can use behavioral change techniques. Identifying individually felt impediments to physical exercise, boosting self-efficacy, effectively setting objectives, preparing for failures, and self-monitoring progress are all helpful tactics.

Illness can rapidly impair a person's physical stability and worsen their walking skills in the elderly. On the other hand, a reduction in physical ability might result in a decline in health and quality of life. Therefore, physical therapy interventions are a crucial part of providing healthcare. There are options to address inactivity, muscle weakness, and certain physical and medical issues through exercise and other therapeutic therapies. The physical therapist can alleviate uncomfortable or dysfunctional symptoms and enhance function using these strategies.

WORKOUT PLANNER

	WEEK 1	WEEK 2	WEEK 3	WEEK 4
MON	Stretching ..... 4 Balance ..... 2 C. Yoga 15	Stretching ..... 12 Balance ..... 12 C. Yoga 43	Stretching ..... 4 Balance ..... 36 C. Yoga 1	Stretching ..... 9 Balance ..... 15 C. Yoga 26
TUES	Stretching ..... 7 Balance ..... 14 C. Yoga 28	Stretching ..... 17 Balance ..... 7 C. Yoga 26	Stretching ..... 1 Balance ..... 6 C. Yoga 44	Stretching ..... 4 Balance ..... 43 C. Yoga 49
WED	Stretching ..... 28 Balance ..... 47 C. Yoga 3	Stretching ..... 28 Balance ..... 8 C. Yoga 22	Stretching ..... 32 Balance ..... 18 C. Yoga 19	Stretching ..... 3 Balance ..... 45 C. Yoga 17
THURS	Stretching ..... 16 Balance ..... 24 C. Yoga 50	Stretching ..... 17 Balance ..... 15 C. Yoga 50	Stretching ..... 31 Balance ..... 16 C. Yoga 5	Stretching ..... 7 Balance ..... 12 C. Yoga 33
FRI	Stretching ..... 18 Balance ..... 39 C. Yoga 41	Stretching ..... 1 Balance ..... 32 C. Yoga 29	Stretching ..... 6 Balance ..... 9 C. Yoga 295	Stretching ..... 4 Balance ..... 9 C. Yoga 35
SAT	Stretching ..... 1 Balance ..... 45 C. Yoga 23	Stretching ..... 30 Balance ..... 31 C. Yoga 11	Stretching ..... 19 Balance ..... 34 C. Yoga 8	Stretching ..... 5 Balance ..... 23 C. Yoga 50

**The numbers indicate the exercises to be performed, for each type of workout
You can start with this work plan. Initially, you can train 10 minutes a day.
Later you can increase the time, considering your physical possibilities.**

Thank you for choosing this book. If you liked it and found it useful, I kindly ask you to leave a review on Amazon, it is very important to me. Thank you!

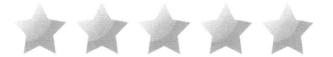

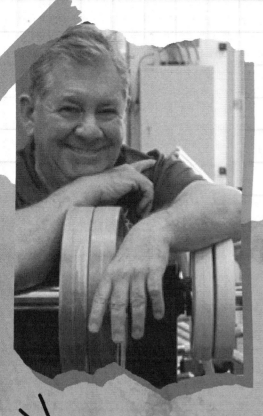

Hi, I'm Daniel

12/11/1962
Zodiac Sign, Scorpio
Height, 183 cm

About me

My name is Daniel Lincoln, and I am a certified instructor and personal trainer. My clients are seniors adults. They always ask me for a simple, quick exercise sheet that they can also do at home to tone muscles and improve balance. I wanted to bring together in this book all the best exercises that will help you feel better and even younger.

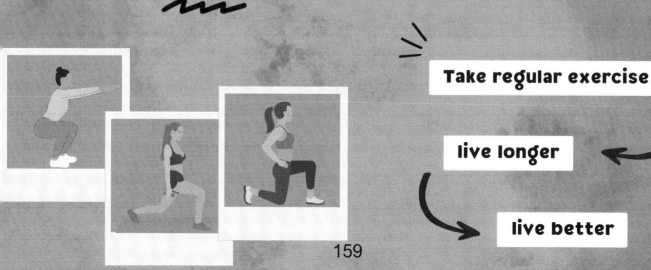

Take regular exercise

live longer

live better

Made in United States
Orlando, FL
09 August 2023

35939681R00087